The One-Pot KETOGENIC DIET Cookbook

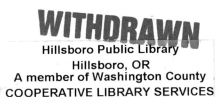

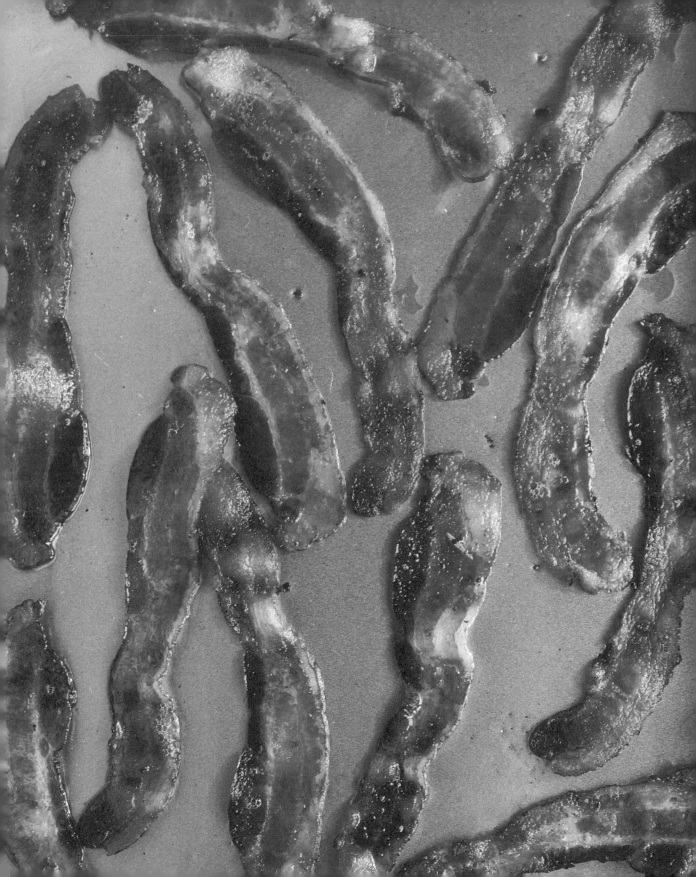

The One-Pot
KETOGENIC DIET
COOKBOOK

100+ EASY WEEKNIGHT MEALS FOR YOUR SKILLET, SLOW COOKER, SHEET PAN, AND MORE

LIZ WILLIAMS

PHOTOGRAPHY BY HÉLÈNE DUJARDIN

ROCKRIDGE
PRESS

For general information on our other products and services or to obtain technical support, please contact our Customer Care Department within the U.S. at (866) 744-2665, or outside the U.S. at (510) 253-0500.

Rockridge Press publishes its books in a variety of electronic and print formats. Some content that appears in print may not be available in electronic books, and vice versa.

TRADEMARKS: Rockridge Press and the Rockridge Press logo are trademarks or registered trademarks of Callisto Media Inc. and/or its affiliates, in the United States and other countries, and may not be used without written permission. All other trademarks are the property of their respective owners. Rockridge Press is not associated with any product or vendor mentioned in this book.

Design by Carol Singer
Photography ©Hélène Dujardin, Food styling by Tami Hardeman

ISBN: Print 978-1-93975-450-9 | eBook 978-1-93975-451-6

33614080738999

For Danny and Gracie Rose

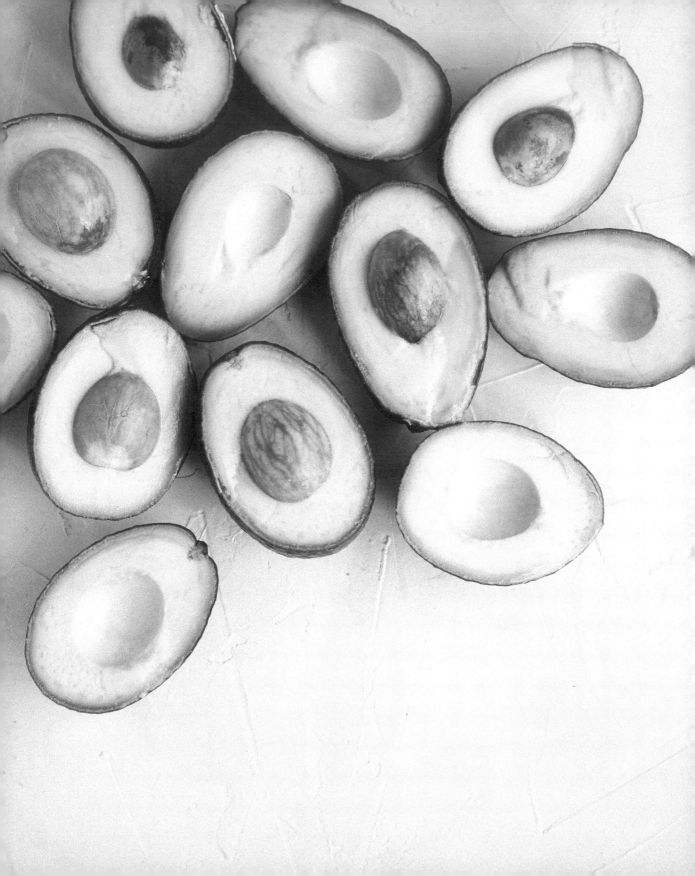

CONTENTS

INTRODUCTION

I know I am not the only one who has struggled to find balance at the dinner table. Life can get so crazy, and figuring out what to make on busy weeknights can sometimes seem impossible—especially if you're trying to follow a diet.

I have spent years and years looking for a quick-fix diet and lifestyle that works for me and my body. Now that I've found it in the ketogenic diet, I want to share it with everyone.

Keto works for my family because we can all eat the same meals and incorporate simple additions if needed. Eliminating the concept that you need to prepare a different dinner for the family is key to your success and sanity when eating keto.

My two-year-old daughter has been eating this way since we introduced solid foods. Now avocados, bacon, and cheese are some of her favorite foods and she's a healthy, growing girl. My husband loves the meals and versatility that keto brings into our lives. Having children (and husbands) eat happily is one of the most important factors in having a positive family mealtime experience.

Through my journey I have learned how to balance and maintain a busy work schedule and life with a toddler, all while keeping everyone fed. My secret: one-pot cooking. Utilizing a single cooking vessel—like a skillet, sheet pan, or slow cooker—to prepare an entire meal simplifies the time I spend in the kitchen cooking, and it also makes clean-up easy. Developing a repertoire of one-pot keto meals has helped me make a commitment to keto every night of the week and helped keep my family fed. It hasn't always been pretty, but I hope you can use what I've learned to find success in your own journey.

Making a plan and being prepared are also important pieces of advice. When I sit down and plan out dinner options for the week, grocery shop, and spend a few hours meal prepping, I'm setting myself up for success. In this book, you'll find the tools for following a ketogenic lifestyle and creating a balanced meal in less time than it would take to load the family up and go out to eat, which will also cut down on your weekly food budget.

When I started my keto lifestyle, I was very overwhelmed with all the information, all the do's and don'ts, and I spent a lot of time wading through it all. I am excited to provide a resource for those who would like to try keto, but want to keep it simple. Having clear, easy-to-follow information is so important. It's tough enough revamping habits we've built over a lifetime, let alone making complicated meals after work. I hope this book will help with a smooth transition into low-carb living.

Within this cookbook you will find easy keto recipes that can be prepared in just one pot or pan, and with familiar ingredients. When I open cookbooks, more often than not, I find recipes with ingredients I'm not sure how to pronounce, let alone find in my local grocery store. Keeping things basic and delicious will keep you on track and able to maintain this lifestyle.

I have seen so many people benefit from living a ketogenic lifestyle. Most, like me, after many failed methods and attempts. I'm so excited to provide a tool that will make becoming healthy a more possible, positive effort for those who want more for themselves and their families.

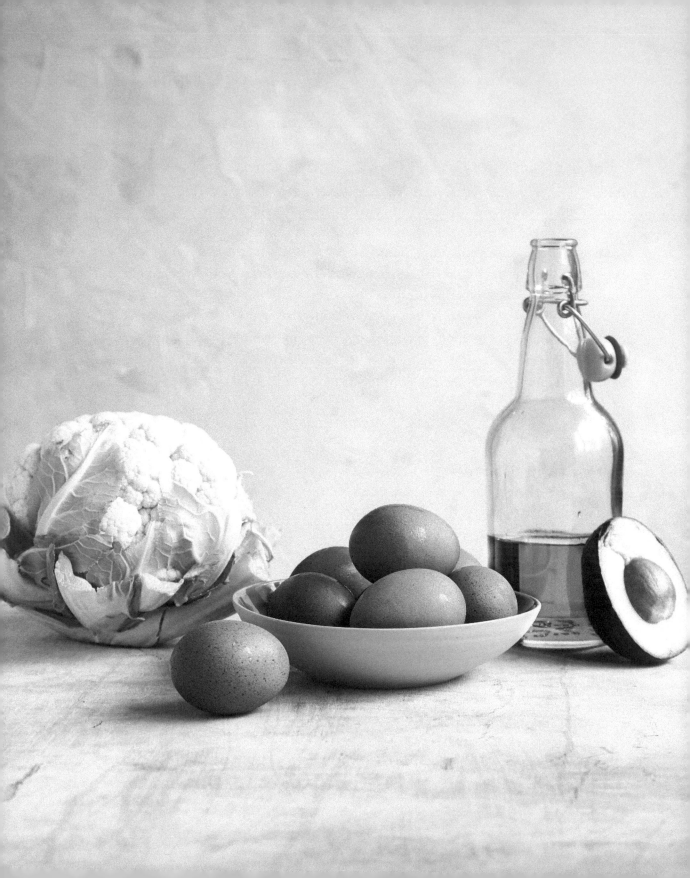

KETO
made EASY

As a working mom, I know how challenging it can be to get a dinner on the table, let alone one that follows a "diet." But I am here to assure you it can be done, even on those crazy weeknights. This chapter will detail the basics of the ketogenic diet and give you the tools you need to transition to and maintain a ketogenic lifestyle, no matter how busy you are.

When I started researching the ketogenic diet, it seemed intimidating, hard to comprehend, and limited. As I studied it, lived it, and felt the benefits, I realized how wrong I was.

Keto became maintainable once I felt comfortable in the aisles of the grocery store and cooking in the kitchen. I know you'll be able to relate, as you gain confidence limiting carbohydrates and incorporating healthy fats into your diet.

Adapting to a ketogenic lifestyle at the dinner table is much easier than it may seem. I hope you'll find ideas and inspiration within these pages to help you find success in maintaining and living a ketogenic lifestyle in your home.

Keto Basics

The ketogenic diet is a low-carb, high-fat, moderate-protein diet that optimizes ketosis. Ketosis is a metabolic process that causes the body (liver) to break down fatty acids into ketone bodies to be used for fuel. When undergoing a ketogenic diet, your body switches from burning mostly carbohydrates for fuel to using fat as its primary fuel source. You are "in ketosis" or "keto-adapted" once your body is metabolizing or burning fat as fuel.

MACRONUTRIENTS

Macronutrients are the three essential components of our diets—fat, protein, and carbohydrates. On a ketogenic diet, 60 to 75 percent of your calories should come from fat, 15 to 30 percent from protein, and 5 to 10 percent from carbohydrates. The goal is to keep your carb intake below 20 to 30 grams per day.

When you first go keto, I strongly encourage you to track your daily macros for the first few weeks, or until you feel comfortable with this new way of eating. I know tracking can seem time-consuming and unrealistic, but it is important to become aware of what your daily macro intake looks like and become familiar with how many carbs are in foods you probably are used to eating every day. Tracking doesn't have to be a lifetime commitment, just until you become more familiar with this lifestyle.

There are tools online that will help you calculate your individual calorie and macronutrient goals. See the Resources section at the end of the book (page 146) for a couple of my favorites. A lot of variables come into play when figuring out your macros, such as your activity level, age, sex, and lean body mass. Ultimately, it's important to experiment and find what ratios your body responds to best.

LOW CARB

On the keto diet, carbohydrates should contribute only 5 to 10 percent of the calories you consume each day. Most people living the keto lifestyle aim for a maximum of 20 to 30 grams of carbs per day. You'll soon discover that carbs add up quickly—to stay at or under the keto ideal of 20 grams of carbs per day, you'll have to severely restrict your diet. One 12-ounce can of Coke, for example, will give you double the daily carb limit allowed on the keto diet.

The carbs you do eat should come from vegetables, nuts, and full-fat dairy products. Refined carbohydrates like grains (bread, pasta, cereals), starch (potatoes, beans, legumes), and fruit are pretty much completely off limits. There are a few exceptions when it comes to fruit, including avocado, which contains lots of the "good fat" that you want to eat on the keto diet, and berries, which can be eaten in moderation.

As you transition into burning fat rather than glucose, you'll realize how much better you feel leaving the starch and grains behind.

MODERATE PROTEIN

Protein should account for between 15 and 30 percent of the calories in your diet.

When you drastically cut your carb intake but continue to eat an unlimited quantity of protein, your body ends up converting that protein into carbohydrates, and then uses that as fuel. In other words, too much protein, no matter how much you limit your carbs, will prevent you from achieving the state of ketosis that makes the keto diet work.

HIGH FAT

Fat is the best part of the keto diet, and it is the glue that holds this lifestyle together. Ideally, 60 to 75 percent of calories should come from fat.

Most of us have been inundated with messages about *reducing* fat in our daily diet for so long that this has become second nature. I still catch myself reaching for fat-free or low-fat products without even thinking. But on a keto diet, you actually want to eat *more* fat. By eating more fat, you encourage your body to use your stored body fat as fuel. This is so cool because it means that donut you ate last year can now be used as energy rather than stored in your hips or thighs.

Because you'll be able to use your stored body fat as energy, you will be hungry less often and you won't dread fasting like you did when burning glucose. As I transitioned into a ketogenic lifestyle, fasting became something I did without thinking about food, and food used to dominate my every thought.

The high-fat aspect of keto is what makes it not only doable, but even enjoyable. Just think, you can eat butter, bacon, avocados, and cheese to your heart's content. And by adding fat to your diet, you'll find that you are hungry less often, you'll have more energy, and your clothes will begin to fit better. The list of benefits from incorporating healthy fats into your diet goes on and on.

WHAT TO EAT

The important part of maintaining a keto lifestyle is keeping things as simple and stress-free as possible. Get rid of the high-carb temptations in your pantry, fridge, and freezer. Commit to a healthy lifestyle for you and for those around you. Go for the low-carb vegetables, healthy oils, full-fat dairy products, and fatty cuts of meat.

Enjoy

It's best to base your diet on whole, unprocessed, single-ingredient foods. Enjoy a variety of meat; fish; eggs; cheeses, butter, cream, and other full-fat dairy products; low-carb nuts, especially pecans, macadamia nuts, brazil nuts, walnuts, almonds, and pine nuts; healthy oils; low-carb condiments; low-carb veggies, like broccoli, cauliflower, and leafy greens—and a whole lot of avocados!

Of course, it's best to buy organic products, but I know that's not always practical in the monthly food budget. Buy the best quality of meats, eggs, dairy products, and vegetables your pocketbook allows.

Watch nutrition labels for hidden sugars and carbs while grocery shopping and cooking. This is especially important when you are buying condiments, sauces, and dressings rather than making them yourself. Store-bought versions of these products are often loaded with sweeteners and starchy thickeners.

Limit

You may enjoy certain higher-carb fruits and vegetables in moderation—a handful of berries or a small serving of squash, carrots, tomatoes, or onions. I cook with a few of these ingredients often, because I love the flavor and texture they bring to my dishes. I feel it's worth using some of my daily carbs to enjoy their contribution.

Watch for higher carbs in cottage cheese, full-fat yogurt, certain nuts—including cashews, chestnuts, and pistachios—and corresponding nut flours. These items are fine to incorporate into your diet in moderation; just be sure to track those carbs!

Avoid

To make things simple, don't eat anything high in carbs. This includes grains, fruit, processed foods, starchy vegetables, sugary drinks, and refined fats. Alcohol should also be avoided, but dry wines and spirits can be consumed in small amounts.

When I first started keto, I missed things like potato chips, homemade comfort food, warm bread, and pasta. I soon found ways to make or adapt high-carb foods, like Vegetable Lasagna (page 84) and Mac 'n' Cheese (page 90), to my low-carb lifestyle, a process I like to call "ketofying."

Fridge and Pantry Staples

When I first started keto, I spent a ton of time figuring out what I could and couldn't eat. I read labels, researched, and made discoveries by trial and error. Here I've compiled what I consider the staples of a ketogenic kitchen.

Avocados. I view avocados as a big part of a ketogenic diet. Not only are they low in carbs, packed full of nutrients, and high in healthy fats, but they also pair well with most dishes and are a great way to add flavor and fat to your diet.

Dairy. Full-fat dairy products, including cream cheese, sour cream, cheeses, heavy (whipping) cream, and grass-fed butter make any dish creamy and rich, and they are keto approved. Avoid dairy products with added sugars, and low-fat and fat-free dairy products.

Eggs. Eggs are convenient, inexpensive, and easy to add to any dish. You can fry, scramble, poach, and hardboil them (page 127). Having a dozen eggs in the fridge at all times is a great way to stay on track and always have a backup meal plan. Half an avocado, bacon, and a couple of fried eggs is the perfect keto meal. Use grass-fed and organic eggs when possible.

Fats & Oils. Olive oil, avocado oil, coconut oil, bacon fat, butter, and ghee are healthy fats that should be incorporated into your diet. Cooking your protein and sautéing your vegetables in these healthy fats makes for satisfying, filling meals and helps you achieve your keto goals. When you are keto-adapted, these healthy fats are your body's primary fuel source, so it's important to incorporate them in your diet.

Meats. When it comes to meats, you have free range—as long as you balance your meals with fatty side dishes when using lean meats. Remember, too much protein is not a good thing, so use protein moderately. Watch for added sugars in bacon and sausages, and stick to uncured and no-sugar-added meats.

Nuts. Nuts and nut butters in moderation are a great fat source. Stick to nuts that are high in fat and low in carbs like almonds, macadamia nuts, walnuts, and pecans. Watch out for pistachios, cashews, and sunflower seeds due to their higher carb content. Nuts are very calorie-dense, so watch your serving size.

Nut Flours. When on a ketogenic diet, almond and coconut flour are great substitutes to use for baking and cooking. Both are gluten-free, grain-free, and low-carb. When making keto-friendly desserts and baked goods or breading protein, it's great to have these flours on hand.

Salt. When living a ketogenic lifestyle, you may experience a decrease in sodium. Adding extra salt to your food may be scary at first, but it is essential when going low-carb. Ideally, use Himalayan salt or sea salt.

Sweeteners. Stevia and erythritol are all-natural sugar replacements. Experiment to see what tastes best to you and what your body responds well to. When you are craving something sweet or need to take your Fat Coffee (page 120) to the next level, it's nice to have these on hand to keep your blood sugar stable. I like Swerve, which is made from erythritol.

Vegetables. When shopping in the produce section, stick to mostly green vegetables. Go for nonstarchy veggies like broccoli (Broccoli-Cheese Soup, page 109), cabbage (Sautéed Cabbage, page 93), cauliflower (Cauliflower Rice, page 128), romaine lettuce (Cobb Salad, page 101), zucchini (Zucchini Noodles, page 129), and Brussels sprouts (Brussels Sprouts with Bacon, page 87). Stay away from starchy vegetables like beans, corn, potatoes, and winter squashes.

Xanthan Gum. Xanthan gum is a great way to thicken gravies, sauces, and soups and stay low carb. A little goes a long way, so start with ¼ teaspoon and go from there. You can buy xanthan gum as a fine powder at any health food store, in the gluten-free section of many supermarkets, or online.

Meal Planning

Prepping for the week ahead is the key to staying on track with your nutritional goals. Meal prep doesn't have to mean cooking your weekend away and destroying the kitchen while you're at it (which may or may not happen on occasion at our house). It simply means prepping a couple of protein options, boiling a dozen eggs, and chopping a variety of veggies for easy, grab-and-go meals and snacks. A few hours of sacrifice on the weekend will lead to a workweek of stress-free, nutritious meals.

Having a plan B and keto-friendly options on hand will prevent dinnertime meltdowns and answer the age-old "what's for dinner" question. I hope I'm not the only one who has burnt the pizza, forgotten the nachos under the broiler, and thought the meat was thawing when it was still frozen solid in the deep freezer. I know there will come a time when you'll appreciate having a backup plan. I recommend making weekend meal prepping a priority so you can stay on track and consistent with your diet.

WEEKLY MENUS

Creating a dinnertime menu for the week ahead is the best way to start meal planning. On Mondays, I like to feel rested, prepared, and ready to crush the list of goals I've made. That happens rarely, but I do my best when I've already prioritized meal prep. Remember, you don't have to have everything in order to live a healthy life. I used that excuse for far too long. Start where you are, with what you have, and invest in a better you.

A few things to keep in mind when you're planning weekly menus:

- Check your local grocery store for current sales.
- Plan for leftovers.
- Set a shopping date and create shopping lists.
- Plan meals where prepped protein can be used throughout the week.

You can follow a ketogenic diet, make it work, and be successful even if you're the only one in the house following this lifestyle. Prepping foods like brown rice, quinoa, and whole-wheat pasta for other members of the household is a great compromise and complements the low-carb meals you'll be making. Keep fresh fruit, veggies, and non-keto snacks stocked for family members. It will take extra willpower on your part to resist indulging in these yourself, but once you start reaping the many benefits of ketosis, the temptation of carbs will be close to nonexistent.

I am often asked how I lost the weight, what the magic pill is, and what the perfect keto macros are. The secret lies in being patient, prepared, and staying consistent. Really, that's the secret. Be prepared.

SHOPPING

After you've mapped out your dinners for the week, make a shopping list. When I go to the store with a plan, it makes it easier to avoid temptations—and the grand total at the end of the shopping trip is usually a little less painful, too. Shop local farmers' markets when possible. And remember to always, always check food labels—those carbs can be very sneaky.

WHAT TO PREP

I have a habit of cooking for a dinner party and not for a family of three. Luckily, my family loves leftovers, and we make good use of them. Taking advantage of leftovers cuts down on waste, eating out, and time spent in the kitchen. Plus, leftovers from last night's dinner make the best breakfast omelets or grab-and-go lunches.

Parboiling in-season vegetables is a great way to cut down on time when it comes to weeknight cooking. To do this, boil water in a large stockpot and blanch the vegetables, cooking them until they are halfway done. Rinse the blanched vegetables with cold water, and drain. You can refrigerate or freeze these prepared vegetables until they are ready to use.

Cooking in large batches and freezing prepped meals, proteins, or sides when possible is another trick I've picked up over the years. I have no shame in admitting one of my prize possessions is our second freezer in the garage. With so much extra space, I have the ability to stock up on good deals, freeze prepped foods, and buy local meat. I know that not everyone has the room to cook in bulk, though.

Chopping or spiralizing raw vegetables ahead and storing them in the fridge can save you time the night of.

Putting together a week's worth of healthy, quick meals can require a fair amount of planning, but it is so worth it when it comes time to put together a weeknight meal.

Let's take a closer look at what weekly meal prep looks like at my house. I've included a sample of five weeknight meals I mapped out for the week, plus a shopping list and details about how I handled the prep. I encourage you to give this one-week meal plan a shot.

In general, I try to keep my shopping list small, planning meals that use some of the same ingredients throughout the week. In the sample weeknight meal plan outlined here, the ham, bacon, broccoli, hardboiled eggs, and mayonnaise are prepped ahead and used in two or more meals. But nothing about this weekly menu feels repetitive.

WEEKLY MENU

MONDAY
Ham, Broccoli, and Mozzarella Frittata (page 27)
Prep ahead: broccoli, ham

TUESDAY
Cobb Salad (page 101)
Prep ahead: Hardboiled Eggs (page 127), ham, Perfectly Cooked Bacon (page 130)

WEDNESDAY
Chicken-Broccoli Curry Bake (page 40)
Prep ahead: chicken, broccoli, Mayonnaise (page 122)

THURSDAY
BLT Lettuce Wraps (page 52)
Prep ahead: Perfectly Cooked Bacon (page 130), Hardboiled Eggs (page 127), Mayonnaise (page 122)

FRIDAY
Cauliflower-Ham Chowder (page 113)
Prep ahead: ham

SHOPPING LIST

Produce

- Avocados, 3
- Broccoli, 3 heads
- Cauliflower, 2 heads
- Cherry tomatoes, 16 ounces
- Lemons, 4
- Romaine lettuce, 4 heads
- Scallions, 3

Meat, Eggs, and Dairy

- Uncured bacon slices, 1 pound
- Blue cheese, crumbled, 1 cup
- Chicken, boneless, skinless breasts, 4 pounds
- Colby-Jack cheese, shredded, 3 cups
- Eggs, large, 14
- Ham, 6 cups diced or cubed
- Heavy (whipping) cream, ½ cup
- Mozzarella cheese, shredded, 2 cups
- Parmesan cheese, grated, ¼ cup
- Sharp white Cheddar cheese, shredded, 2 cups
- Sour cream, 1 pint (always use the full-fat variety)

Fats & Oils

- Olive oil

Pantry Items

- Apple cider vinegar
- Chicken broth, 3 cups
- Dijon mustard
- Sugar substitute (such as Swerve)

Herbs & Spices

- Bay leaf
- Curry powder
- Garlic salt
- Onion powder
- Pepper
- Salt

SUNDAY PREP LIST

1. Hardboil a dozen eggs (see Hardboiled Eggs, page 127).

2. Cook a pound of bacon for the week (see Perfectly Cooked Bacon, page 130).

3. Cook 4 pounds boneless, skinless chicken breasts: Place whole boneless, skinless chicken breasts in a slow cooker and season with salt and pepper. Cook on low for 6 to 8 hours, or until the chicken is cooked through. Remove the chicken from the slow cooker and let rest for 10 to 15 minutes. Shred the chicken using 2 forks, and then return the shredded meat to the slow cooker with the juices. Divide into meal-sized portions and store in airtight containers in the refrigerator for up to 4 days (or in the freezer for up to 3 months).

4. Make Mayonnaise (page 122).

5. Wash and prep a variety of vegetables for easy salads and low-carb snacks.

6. Blanch fresh broccoli (see page 9), and store it in an airtight container in the refrigerator.

START PLANNING!

Now it's your turn! Use the following blank menu and shopping list to plan a week's worth of weeknight keto meals. After some time, you'll start to develop your own tips and tricks.

WEEKLY MENU

MONDAY

TUESDAY

WEDNESDAY

THURSDAY

FRIDAY

SHOPPING LIST

PRODUCE

FATS & OILS

MEAT, EGGS & DAIRY

PANTRY ITEMS

HERBS & SPICES

THROW-TOGETHER KETO COMBOS

As you become increasingly familiar with the ins and outs of keto, you'll find meal and grocery list planning to be less stressful and time-consuming. Having a few low-carb basics around at all times will keep you on track and burning fat. Use the formula of a base + protein + fat to whip up quick keto meals in no time.

Pick a base

- Bed of spinach
- Chopped romaine lettuce
- Cauliflower Rice (page 128)
- Broth or Bone Broth (page 121)
- Sautéed Cabbage (page 93)
- Steamed broccoli florets

Pick a protein

- Uncured bacon
- Chicken drumsticks
- Ground beef (80% protein / 20% fat)
- Sausage
- Canned tuna
- Smoked salmon

Pick a fat

- Half avocado
- 2 slices or ¼ cup shredded cheese
- 2 tablespoons low-carb salad dressing
- 2 tablespoons Mayonnaise (page 122)
- 2 tablespoons sour cream or heavy (whipping) cream
- Fried egg or Hardboiled Egg (page 127)

One-Pot Cooking

The recipes in this book were created to demonstrate that a high-fat, low-carb diet can be simple, made with familiar, everyday ingredients, and keep the dinner cleanup to a minimum.

When I put a beautiful meal on the dinner table in my early cooking days, my kitchen was left a disaster, the sink overflowing with pots and pans. Once I discovered the convenience and potential of one-pot cooking, dinnertime became a lot more enjoyable and convenient for the whole family. When I transitioned to a keto diet, I still relied on one-pot meals, especially when it came to weeknight cooking.

One-pot cooking is not just for the easy cleanup. When a meal is all in one pot or pan, the flavors have a chance to marinate and blend with one another. This is a great way to have a delicious, quick, streamlined meal without ending up with a pile of dishes. It also helps to keep ingredient lists and prep times short.

All the recipes in this book use only one of the pieces of kitchen equipment outlined below—or none at all. Icons on each recipe will tell you what the recipe requires. The two chapters where you'll find exceptions are Keto Basics and Sweets (chapters 9 and 10), but even these recipes keep the required cooking equipment to a minimum.

 Casserole dish or baking dish. Being able to throw everything into a baking dish and into the oven is priceless and fuss-free. There are no boundaries when it comes to baking in a casserole dish, plus it makes it easy to store precooked meals in the freezer.

 Cast iron or other skillet. This has been a favorite of mine since I watched my grandmother and grandfather cook only with cast iron in the kitchen. Cast iron is so versatile and can go from the stovetop to the oven or even the barbecue, which makes it ideal for one-pan cooking. What makes cast iron cookware so great is the easy cleanup and seasoning of your cookware, which, if done correctly, makes it a chemical-free nonstick option. When you are finished using your skillet, clean it, coat it lightly with oil, and then heat it for several minutes before storing.

Muffin tin. Muffin tins are far more versatile than you might think, great for sweet and savory foods alike. I love to use my muffin tins to create grab-and-go breakfasts that are easy to make ahead, and single-serving desserts.

 Sheet pan. My favorite thing about a sheet pan is being able to line and cover it with aluminum foil or parchment paper for easy cleanup and leftover storage. This takes one-pan cooking to a new level. The sky is the limit with a sheet pan; get creative and keep things simple for dinnertime.

 Slow cooker. Slow cooking may be my personal favorite because of the ease and one-step preparation. There is nothing like throwing a bunch of ingredients into the slow cooker before work and coming home to the smell of a home-cooked meal with no stress. I have recently discovered slow-cooker liners, which make cleanup even easier.

 Stockpot or Dutch oven. There is so much potential when it comes to one-pot cooking in a Dutch oven or stockpot. You can steam, sauté, simmer, braise, and roast stress-free and with minimal cleanup.

About the Recipes

Living the keto lifestyle does not need to be complex and intimidating. I am here to show you how easy it can be to maintain a low-carb, high-fat diet. My goal is to give you the tools to transition from a diet heavy in carbs to one that is low in carbs, high in fat, and totally satisfying—even with a hectic schedule.

With that in mind, the recipes you'll find here are all designed to fit with the keto lifestyle, while still being easy enough to whip up on a busy weeknight. These recipes are all cooked in one pot or pan (or not cooked at all), and they have short lists of easy-to-find, familiar ingredients. Most can be cooked in 45 minutes or less, many in under 30 minutes.

Each recipe includes several features to help you navigate the book as easily as possible:

• Number of servings, prep time, and cooking time are listed at the top of each recipe.

• An icon illustrates what cooking vessel is needed—casserole dish or baking dish, cast iron skillet, muffin tin, sheet pan, slow cooker, stockpot or Dutch oven.

• Recipe labels show, at a glance, which recipes are Dairy-Free, Nut-Free, Egg-Free, Paleo, Vegetarian, and/or can be made in Under 30 Minutes. All the recipes in this book are gluten-free.

• Recipe tips offer suggestions for recipe alterations that can make the dish free of the top eight allergens or Paleo-friendly and feature ideas for changing up the dishes to add variety to your meals, suggestions for making the dish ahead of time, and advice on shopping for and prepping ingredients that you might not be familiar with.

• Macro percentages and complete nutritional information are included for each recipe to help you stay on track with your goals.

KETO COOKING TIPS

Stock up. Fill your fridge, pantry, and kitchen with frequently used ingredients, spices, kitchen gadgets, and sharp knives.

Look for in-season produce. Whenever possible, buy seasonal produce—it saves money, tastes great, and is more widely available than out-of-season produce.

Prep ahead. Precook meats like ground beef, bacon, and chicken breasts for convenient additions to vegetable dishes and salads. Wash, trim, and chop or even partially cook vegetables ahead of time, too.

Slow cook. Take advantage of the set-and-go feature on your slow cooker for a stress-free weeknight meal.

Go from stovetop to oven in one pan. Invest in a cast iron skillet that can go from burner to oven to make it even easier to make one-pan meals.

Purée right in the pot. With an immersion blender, you can purée soups and sauces right in the pot they're cooked in, making for easy cleanup. Immersion blenders are also useful for whipping cream and making frothy Fat Coffee (page 120) without a blender.

Turn your veggies into noodles. One of my favorite gadgets in the kitchen is a spiralizer, which turns vegetables into noodle-like strands. If you don't have a spiralizer, a mandolin or vegetable peeler will work, too.

Add avocado. Whenever you have a dish that doesn't meet your fat needs, add half an avocado. It will add flavor, texture, and depth to just about any dish, as well as add the healthy fats you need.

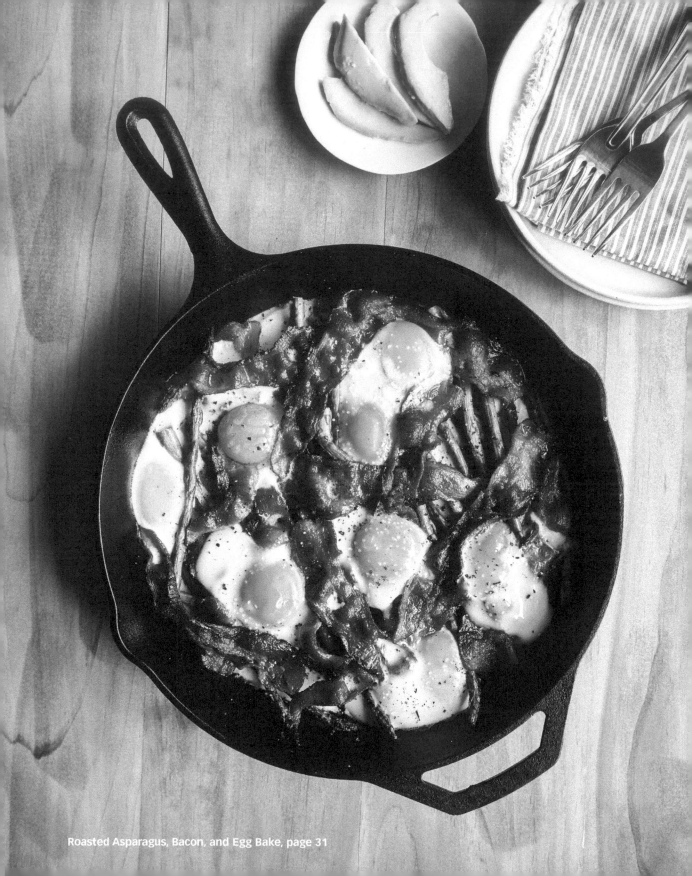

Roasted Asparagus, Bacon, and Egg Bake, page 31

CHAPTER 2

EGGS *for* DINNER

Avocado Egg Salad

If you prepped hardboiled eggs for the week, this recipe is done and on your plate in 5 minutes or less. This flavorful egg salad is great wrapped in lettuce, on its own, or even over a green salad—you won't even need dressing! Punch up your keto egg salad even more by adding diced pickles, celery, or scallions for some crunch. Adding Mayonnaise (page 122) will give the egg salad a creamier texture.

Serves 4

Prep time | 5 minutes

DAIRY-FREE, NUT-FREE, PALEO, VEGETARIAN, UNDER 30 MINUTES

2 avocados, pitted, divided

6 Hardboiled Eggs (page 127), peeled, divided

1 teaspoon prepared mustard

1 tablespoon freshly squeezed lemon juice

1 tablespoon apple cider vinegar

½ teaspoon paprika

1 teaspoon garlic powder

Salt

Freshly ground black pepper

Leafy greens or romaine lettuce leaves, for serving

1. In a medium bowl, mash 1 of the avocados with the yolks of 3 of the eggs and the mustard, lemon juice, vinegar, paprika, and garlic powder.

2. Roughly chop the egg yolks and whites of the remaining 3 eggs, and add them to the yolk and avocado mixture.

3. Dice the remaining avocado, and stir it into the mixture. Season with salt and pepper.

4. Serve immediately over greens or in a lettuce wrap.

MAKE AHEAD *Although this salad is best eaten the day it is made, it will keep, covered in the refrigerator, for up to 3 days.*

MACRONUTRIENTS **70% FAT,** 16% PROTEIN, 14% CARBS

PER SERVING Calories: 259; Total Fat: 21g; Saturated Fat: 4g; Protein: 11g; Total Carbs: 10g; Fiber: 6g; Net Carbs: 4g; Cholesterol: 279mg

Cream Cheese and Avocado Scramble

Before I started living low carb, I had never heard of cream cheese in scrambled eggs, and man had I been missing out. Scrambled eggs don't have to be boring and dry. They can be so delicate, rich, and creamy that you'll never tire of eating them.

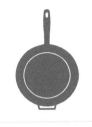

Serves 4

Prep time | 5 minutes   *Cook time* | 10 minutes

NUT-FREE, VEGETARIAN, UNDER 30 MINUTES

8 large eggs

2 tablespoons heavy (whipping) cream

Pinch salt

Pinch freshly ground black pepper

2 tablespoons salted butter

¼ cup cream cheese

½ cup shredded Cheddar cheese or Monterey Jack

2 avocados, sliced

1. In a medium mixing bowl, whisk together the eggs, cream, salt, and pepper until smooth.

2. In a large skillet over medium heat, melt the butter. Add the egg mixture and cook, stirring in a figure-eight motion, for about 4 minutes, until the eggs are about halfway cooked.

3. Add the cream cheese and shredded cheese, and stir gently. Cook until your desired consistency.

4. Serve immediately, topped with the sliced avocado.

VARIATION TIP *Try adding cubed ham and chives to your cream cheese scrambled eggs.*

MACRONUTRIENTS **77% FAT,** 15% PROTEIN, 8% CARBS

PER SERVING Calories: 444; Total Fat: 38g; Saturated Fat: 15g; Protein: 18g; Total Carbs: 9g; Fiber: 6g; Net Carbs: 3g; Cholesterol: 416mg

English Breakfast

So, what does a typical English breakfast consist of? Traditionally, a full English breakfast includes two sausages, three rashers of bacon, fried eggs, fried sliced tomatoes, and lashings of mushrooms with black pudding, which makes for an almost perfect keto meal. I've replaced the black pudding and tomatoes with creamy avocado.

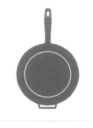

Serves 4

Prep time | 5 minutes   *Cook time* | 20 minutes

DAIRY-FREE, NUT-FREE, PALEO, UNDER 30 MINUTES

4 large eggs

8 uncured bacon slices

4 sausage links

2 cups sliced mushrooms

2 avocados, sliced

Salt

Freshly ground black pepper

1. In a large skillet, cook the eggs to your liking: scrambled, fried, poached, etc. Remove from the pan and set aside.

2. In the same skillet over medium heat, cook the bacon and sausage links for 8 to 10 minutes, until browned. Transfer to a paper towel-lined plate.

3. Add the sliced mushrooms to the rendered bacon and sausage fat in the pan. Cook, stirring constantly, for 5 to 6 minutes, or until the mushrooms are softened and browned.

4. Arrange the eggs, bacon, sausage, mushrooms, and avocado on a plate. Season with salt and pepper and serve immediately.

ALLERGEN TIP *In place of the eggs, sauté 4 cups of fresh spinach in the bacon and sausage fat with the mushrooms.*

MACRONUTRIENTS **75% FAT,** 16% PROTEIN, 9% CARBS

PER SERVING Calories: 404; Total Fat: 34g; Saturated Fat: 10g; Protein: 17g; Total Carbs: 9g; Fiber: 6g; Net Carbs: 4g; Cholesterol: 674mg

Eggs Benedict Cups

These delicious bacon cups are the perfect thing to make in advance. Sometimes I'll double this recipe and store the extra cups for later. If you like your bacon crispy like I do, place the muffin tin in the oven for 5 to 10 minutes before you crack the eggs over it. The cooked cups can be stored in an airtight container for up to 5 days. Reheat them for 30 to 60 seconds in the microwave.

Serves 6

Prep time | 10 minutes   *Cook time* | 20 minutes

NUT-FREE, UNDER 30 MINUTES

Cooking spray, salted butter, or olive oil, for preparing the pan

12 uncured bacon or Canadian bacon slices

12 large eggs

½ cup shredded Colby-Jack or mozzarella cheese

Salt

Freshly ground black pepper

Hollandaise Sauce (page 125)

1. Preheat the oven to 350°F. Coat a 12-cup muffin tin with cooking spray.

2. Line each muffin cup with 1 slice of bacon. Crack one egg into each muffin cup. Sprinkle the cheese over the top, and season with salt and pepper.

3. Bake for 15 to 20 minutes, or until the eggs have reached your desired doneness.

4. Serve hot with hollandaise sauce spooned over each cup.

VARIATION TIP *You can add your favorite low-carb veggies before you crack the egg into the bacon cup and bake.*

MAKE IT PALEO *Leave out the cheese and use the dairy-free Hollandaise Sauce variation (page 125).*

MACRONUTRIENTS **63% FAT**, 26% PROTEIN, 11% CARBS

PER SERVING Calories: 369; Total Fat: 26g; Saturated Fat: 13g; Protein: 25g; Total Carbs: 11g; Fiber: 0g; Net Carbs: 11g; Cholesterol: 433mg

Crustless Dinner Quiche

I love the versatility of this dish. The recipe outlined here makes a delicious egg dinner, but you can have it for breakfast, too. The options are endless as far as what you can add to quiche. If you have any leftovers, they can be turned into a great breakfast by whisking them with eggs, cheese, and cream. Add a few slices of bacon and a cup of coffee, and you're good to go. Who said keto can't be easy?

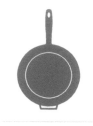

Serves 6

Prep time | 10 minutes, plus 10 minutes to stand   *Cook time* | 30 minutes

NUT-FREE, VEGETARIAN

2 tablespoons salted butter, for preparing the pan

6 large eggs

1 cup heavy (whipping) cream

1½ cups shredded Muenster or Colby-Jack cheese

Salt

Freshly ground black pepper

8 ounces frozen chopped spinach, thawed and squeezed dry

1. Preheat the oven to 375°F. Grease a large, cast iron skillet with the butter.

2. In a medium bowl, whisk together the eggs, cream, and cheese, and season with salt and pepper. Add the drained spinach to the mixture, and stir to blend.

3. Pour the mixture into the prepared skillet.

4. Bake for 30 minutes, or until the eggs have set.

5. Let stand for 10 minutes and serve.

VARIATION TIP *You can use fresh spinach, but you'll have to cook down 3 bunches to equal 1 (8-ounce) package of frozen spinach. This book is all about easy meals, though, and you can't beat frozen spinach for efficiency.*

MACRONUTRIENTS **79% FAT,** 17% PROTEIN, 4% CARBS

PER SERVING Calories: 332; Total Fat: 29g; Saturated Fat: 19g; Protein: 13g; Total Carbs: 3g; Fiber: 1g; Net Carbs: 2g; Cholesterol: 272mg

Ham, Broccoli, and Mozzarella Frittata

A frittata is a very keto, cost-effective Italian dish. It also happens to make for some awesome leftovers. Traditionally, frittatas are round because they are baked in a cast iron skillet, but if you're using a baking dish instead, as I do, square ones taste just as good.

Serves 6

Prep time | 10 minutes   *Cook time* | 30 minutes

NUT-FREE

Olive oil cooking spray

5 cups small broccoli florets, blanched for 2 minutes (see page 9), then drained well

1 cup diced ham

2 cups shredded mozzarella cheese

8 large eggs, beaten

Salt

Freshly ground black pepper

Sour cream, for serving (optional)

1. Preheat the oven to 375°F. Spray a 9-by-13-inch baking dish with the cooking spray.

2. Layer the broccoli, ham, and mozzarella in the prepared baking dish.

3. Season the eggs with salt and pepper and pour over the top of the ingredients in the baking dish. Stir everything together with a fork.

4. Bake for 25 to 30 minutes, or until the top is just lightly browned (a golden top means the center is overcooked).

5. Serve warm, topped with sour cream (if using).

MAKE IT PALEO *Replace the shredded mozzarella cheese with 2 cups of fresh spinach leaves and leave out the optional sour cream.*

MACRONUTRIENTS **52% FAT**, 39% PROTEIN, 9% CARBS

PER SERVING Calories: 274; Total Fat: 16g; Saturated Fat: 6g; Protein: 27g; Total Carbs: 6g; Fiber: 2g; Net Carbs: 4g; Cholesterol: 282mg

Slow Cooker Omelet

This breakfast casserole slow cooker recipe takes the hassle out of weeknight cooking. Toss all the ingredients into the slow cooker, set it, and forget all about it until dinnertime. You could top this fluffy egg casserole with sour cream, hot sauce, avocado, or salsa.

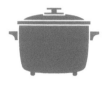

Serves 8

Prep time | 20 minutes   *Cook time* | 6 hours
NUT-FREE

Olive oil cooking spray (optional)

2 cups broccoli or cauliflower florets, chopped, divided

1 green bell pepper, seeded and diced, divided

1 yellow onion, diced, divided

1 pound breakfast sausage, browned and crumbled, divided

2 cups shredded Cheddar or Colby cheese, divided

12 large eggs, beaten

1 cup heavy (whipping) cream

Pinch salt

Pinch freshly ground black pepper

1. Spray a slow cooker with the cooking spray or line it with a slow-cooker liner.

2. Layer about half of the broccoli, bell pepper, onion, sausage, and cheese in the slow cooker. Repeat layering with the remaining ingredients.

3. In a large mixing bowl, whisk together the eggs, cream, salt, and pepper. Pour the egg mixture over the layered ingredients in the slow cooker.

4. Cover and cook on low for 5 to 6 hours, until the casserole is browned around the edges.

5. Serve hot.

MAKE AHEAD *This is a great recipe to prepare ahead of time, cut into single servings, and store refrigerated in an airtight container or resealable plastic bag. Warm it up in the microwave at work or enjoy an easy breakfast at the campsite.*

MACRONUTRIENTS **74% FAT,** 20% PROTEIN, 6% CARBS

PER SERVING Calories: 519; Total Fat: 43g; Saturated Fat: 20g; Protein: 26g; Total Carbs: 6g; Fiber: 1g; Net Carbs: 5g; Cholesterol: 378mg

Mexican Hash

Spicy chorizo sausage gives this quick-and-easy hash loads of flavor. Topped with scrambled, fried, or poached eggs and creamy avocado, it makes for a satisfying weeknight dinner. For even more flavor, add sour cream and/or hot sauce.

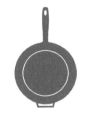

Prep time | 10 minutes   *Cook time* | 25 minutes

DAIRY-FREE, NUT-FREE, PALEO

Serves 4

4 large eggs

2 tablespoons olive oil

1 yellow onion, diced

1 green bell pepper, seeded and diced

1 zucchini, chopped

1 tomato, chopped

12 ounces chorizo, casing removed

2 cups fresh spinach

Salt

Freshly ground black pepper

1 avocado, diced

1. In a large skillet, cook the eggs to your liking: scrambled, fried, poached, etc. Remove from the pan and set aside.

2. In the same skillet over medium heat, heat the olive oil. Add the onion and green pepper and cook, stirring constantly, for 4 to 5 minutes, or until the onion is translucent. Add the zucchini and tomato and cook, stirring occasionally, for 5 more minutes.

3. Add the chorizo to the skillet and cook, stirring, for an additional 5 minutes. Add the spinach and cook until it starts to wilt, 1 to 2 more minutes. Season with salt and pepper.

4. Serve hot, topped with the eggs and avocado.

ALLERGEN TIP *Skip the eggs and double up on avocado to keep your macros in range.*

MACRONUTRIENTS **71% FAT**, 20% PROTEIN, 9% CARBS

PER SERVING Calories: 569; Total Fat: 45g; Saturated Fat: 15g; Protein: 29g; Total Carbs: 11g; Fiber: 2g; Net Carbs: 9g; Cholesterol: 261mg

Upgraded Scrambled Eggs and Bacon

This dish is based on the classic breakfast combo of eggs and bacon. With a few additions, it makes for a satisfying yet easy dinner. Remember, it's best to bring your eggs to room temperature before cooking. When you take the skillet off the heat, you'll want the eggs to be slightly runny. The eggs will continue to cook after they are removed from the heat source.

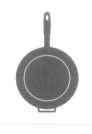

Serves 4

Prep time | 5 minutes   *Cook time* | 20 minutes

NUT-FREE, UNDER 30 MINUTES

8 uncured bacon slices

8 large eggs

¼ cup heavy (whipping) cream

¼ cup ricotta cheese

¼ cup minced chives or scallions

1 avocado, sliced

Salt

Freshly ground black pepper

1. Lay the bacon slices in a large, cold skillet. Set over medium-low heat and cook until the bacon reaches your desired crispiness, about 8 minutes. Transfer the bacon to a paper towel–lined plate.

2. Pour off and discard most of the bacon grease, but leave enough to coat the bottom of the skillet.

3. In a medium bowl, lightly whisk the eggs, cream, cheese, and chives together.

4. Return the skillet to the stove over low heat. Add the egg mixture to the hot pan and cook, stirring gently with a spatula, for 5 to 8 minutes.

5. Season the eggs with salt and pepper, and serve immediately with the reserved bacon and the avocado slices.

MAKE IT PALEO *Substitute coconut milk for the cream and ¼ cup fresh spinach for the ricotta.*

MACRONUTRIENTS **80% FAT,** 17% PROTEIN, 3% CARBS

PER SERVING Calories: 535; Total Fat: 48g; Saturated Fat: 17g; Protein: 22g; Total Carbs: 5g; Fiber: 2g; Net Carbs: 3g; Cholesterol: 498mg

Roasted Asparagus, Bacon, and Egg Bake

This is a complete meal with eggs, crispy bacon, and oven-roasted asparagus in just one skillet. If you are short on time and want to skip a step in this recipe, use a sheet pan instead of a skillet. Lay out the prepped asparagus on the pan, place the raw bacon on top of the spears, and season with salt and pepper. Bake for 12 to 15 minutes, or until the bacon is almost crisp. Remove the pan from the oven and toss the bacon and asparagus. Crack the eggs over the top and bake until the eggs reach your desired doneness, about 5 to 7 minutes. Serve with the sliced avocado.

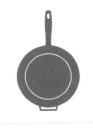

Serves 4

Prep time | **5 minutes**   *Cook time* | **20 minutes**

DAIRY-FREE, NUT-FREE, PALEO, UNDER 30 MINUTES

12 uncured bacon slices

16 to 20 asparagus spears, ends snapped off and discarded

Salt

Freshly ground black pepper

8 large eggs

1 avocado, sliced

1. Preheat the oven to 425°F.

2. In large cast iron skillet over medium heat, cook the bacon. Turn the slices with tongs every few minutes and cook until the bacon is 75% cooked, 5 to 7 minutes. Transfer to a paper towel–lined plate.

3. Drain the bacon grease from the skillet and discard, leaving 3 tablespoons of bacon fat in the pan. Add the trimmed asparagus spears to the skillet, season with salt and pepper, and toss until coated with fat.

4. Bake in the oven for 6 to 8 minutes, or until the spears start to soften. Remove from the oven and turn the asparagus with tongs. Return the bacon to the skillet. Crack the eggs over the top of the bacon and asparagus.

5. Return the skillet to the oven and bake for 5 to 7 minutes, or until the eggs reach desired doneness.

6. Serve immediately with the avocado slices.

Continued

Roasted Asparagus, Bacon, and Egg Bake *Continued*

VARIATION TIP *Replace the asparagus with halved Brussels sprouts. Prepare them just like the asparagus, but the Brussels sprouts may need to bake for an additional few minutes before adding the bacon and eggs to the skillet. Another option would be adding halved cherry tomatoes prior to baking and topping the skillet with balsamic vinegar, fresh basil, and mozzarella cheese.*

MACRONUTRIENTS **66% FAT,** 25% PROTEIN, 9% CARBS

PER SERVING Calories: 370; Total Fat: 27g; Saturated Fat: 8g; Protein: 23g; Total Carbs: 8g; Fiber: 5g; Net Carbs: 3g; Cholesterol: 394mg

Pizza Frittata

Who needs pizza crust when you've got this tasty frittata that has all the flavors you love in pizza without all the carbs? You can swap out the pepperoni for your favorite pizza topping, such as cooked Italian sausage or ham.

Prep time | 10 minutes   *Cook time* | 15 minutes

NUT-FREE, UNDER 30 MINUTES

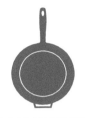

Serves 4

2 tablespoons unsalted butter

1 cup sliced mushrooms

¼ red onion, chopped

6 ounces mini pepperoni (or chopped pepperoni)

6 eggs, beaten

2 tablespoons tomato paste

1 teaspoon dried oregano

1 teaspoon garlic powder

½ cup grated mozzarella cheese, or 4 ounces sliced fresh mozzarella

1. Preheat your oven's broiler on high heat and adjust the oven rack to the upper level.

2. In a large skillet, heat the butter on medium-high until it bubbles.

3. Add the mushrooms and onion and cook until the vegetables are soft, about five minutes. Add the pepperoni and cook 1 minute more.

4. In a bowl, whisk together the eggs, tomato paste, oregano, and garlic powder.

5. Carefully add the egg mixture to the skillet. Allow the eggs to set on the bottom. Using a spatula, carefully pull the set eggs away from the side of the pan, tilt the pan, and allow uncooked eggs to run to fill the edges. Cook until the eggs are set completely.

6. Sprinkle the cheese on top of the eggs. Place in the oven and broil until the frittata puffs and the cheese melts and browns slightly, three to five minutes.

7. Cut into wedges to serve.

TIP *You can also use bacon in place of the pepperoni. If you use regular bacon, omit the butter and cut the bacon into pieces. Brown the bacon first and then use the bacon fat to cook the vegetables.*

MACRONUTRIENTS **74% FAT**, 22% PROTEIN, 4% CARBS

PER SERVING Calories: 421; Total Fat: 35g; Saturated Fat: 14g; Protein: 23g; Total Carbs: 4g; Fiber: 1g; Net Carbs: 3g; Cholesterol: 387mg

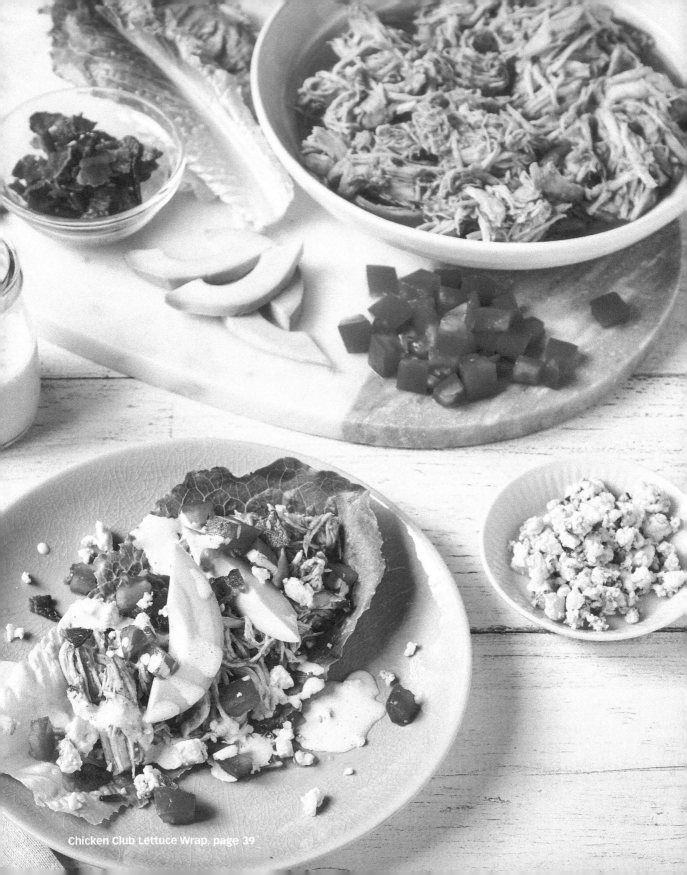

Chicken Club Lettuce Wrap, page 39

CHAPTER

3

CHICKEN

Chicken Fajita Skillet

This dish is a staple at my house and keeps me on track with my ketogenic lifestyle. Fajitas are super versatile. You can substitute any protein of your choice for the chicken or mix in some other veggies, for instance. It's a quick and easy weeknight meal that everyone will love.

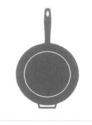

Serves 4

Prep time | 10 minutes   *Cook time* | 20 minutes

NUT-FREE, EGG-FREE

FOR THE FAJITAS

1 pound boneless, skinless chicken breasts, sliced

3 tablespoons olive oil, divided

¼ cup chopped cilantro leaves

1 garlic clove, minced

1 teaspoon ground cumin

1 teaspoon salt, plus additional as needed

2 bell peppers, seeded and thinly sliced

1 yellow onion, thinly sliced

Freshly ground black pepper

FOR SERVING

1 cup sour cream

1 avocado, sliced

1 cup shredded Cheddar or Monterey Jack cheese

1. In large bowl, combine the sliced chicken breast and 1 tablespoon of olive oil with the cilantro, garlic, cumin, and salt. Toss until the chicken is coated.

2. In a large skillet over medium heat, heat 1 tablespoon of olive oil. Add the bell peppers and onion and cook, stirring occasionally, until they are lightly browned and the onion is soft, 5 to 7 minutes. Transfer the mixture to a paper towel–lined plate and set aside.

3. In the same skillet over medium heat, cook the chicken mixture, stirring occasionally, until the chicken is cooked through, 8 to 12 minutes.

4. Return the sautéed onion and bell peppers to the skillet, and heat until sizzling. Season with salt and pepper.

5. Serve the chicken fajitas hot, topped with the sour cream, avocado slices, and cheese.

VARIATION TIP *You can make this dish with just about any protein you like. Try substituting thinly sliced beef, pork, or lamb.*

MACRONUTRIENTS **63% FAT,** 26% PROTEIN, 11% CARBS

PER SERVING Calories: 522; Total Fat: 37g; Saturated Fat: 16g; Protein: 35g; Total Carbs: 15g; Fiber: 5g; Net Carbs: 10g; Cholesterol: 111mg

Cauliflower Rice and Chicken Drumsticks

This is one of the very first recipes I wrote, and to this day it is still one of my family's favorites. If cauliflower isn't frequently used at your house, it needs to be! It's the perfect substitute for those high-carb veggies, like potatoes and winter squash, when living a low-carb lifestyle.

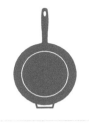

Serves 3

Prep time | 5 minutes   *Cook time* | 30 minutes

NUT-FREE, EGG-FREE

4 tablespoons salted butter, divided

1 yellow onion, chopped

3 cups Cauliflower Rice (page 128)

½ cup heavy (whipping) cream or full-fat coconut milk

½ cup shredded Cheddar cheese

Pinch salt

Pinch freshly ground black pepper

6 chicken drumsticks

1 tablespoon onion powder

1 tablespoon garlic salt

1. In a large skillet over medium heat, melt 2 tablespoons of butter. Add the onion and cook, stirring occasionally, until it is soft and translucent, about 5 minutes. Add the cauliflower rice and continue to cook for 5 minutes more. Add the cream, cheese, salt, and pepper, and stir until the cheese is melted. Transfer the mixture to a medium bowl and set aside.

2. Melt the remaining 2 tablespoons of butter in the same skillet over medium heat. Season the drumsticks with the onion powder, garlic, salt, and pepper. Cook the drumsticks, turning them frequently, until the skin is golden brown and the chicken is cooked through, about 15 minutes.

3. Serve the drumsticks immediately with the cauliflower rice on the side.

VARIATION TIP *You can change the flavor of this recipe up by using different cheeses. Try substituting pepper Jack or another flavorful cheese for the Cheddar.*

MACRONUTRIENTS **70% FAT,** 22% PROTEIN, 8% CARBS

PER SERVING Calories: 621; Total Fat: 48g; Saturated Fat: 28g; Protein: 32g; Total Carbs: 11g; Fiber: 3g; Net Carbs: 8g; Cholesterol: 202mg

Chicken Cordon Bleu Casserole

This deconstructed version of a traditional French classic dish is one that the whole family will enjoy. Save any leftovers for the next day's breakfast. Reheated and paired with eggs, this casserole is a great way to start your morning.

Prep time | 10 minutes, plus 5 minutes to rest   *Cook time* | 30 minutes

NUT FREE, EGG-FREE

Serves 8

1 cup (2 sticks) salted butter, melted, plus 2 tablespoons for preparing the baking dish

4 cups cooked, shredded chicken breast (see page 12)

1 cup diced ham

1 cup cream cheese, at room temperature

1 tablespoon Dijon mustard

2 tablespoons freshly squeezed lemon juice

Pinch salt

Pinch freshly ground black pepper

2 cups shredded Swiss cheese

1. Preheat the oven to 350°F. Grease a 9-by-13-inch baking dish with 2 tablespoons of butter.

2. Layer the shredded chicken and ham in the prepared baking dish.

3. In a small bowl, whisk together the melted butter, cream cheese, mustard, lemon juice, salt, and pepper. Spread the mixture over the top of the chicken and ham in the baking dish. Sprinkle the Swiss cheese over the top.

4. Bake for 30 minutes, or until the casserole is heated throughout and the cheese is browned.

5. Let rest for 5 minutes and serve hot.

MAKE AHEAD *This is a great recipe to double: make one for dinner and another to stash in the freezer for another day. Cover the unbaked casserole with aluminum foil and freeze. Thaw the casserole in the refrigerator overnight, and then follow the baking instructions above.*

MACRONUTRIENTS **72% FAT,** 27% PROTEIN, 1% CARBS

PER SERVING Calories: 587; Total Fat: 47g; Saturated Fat: 4g; Protein: 39g; Total Carbs: 2g; Fiber: 0g; Net Carbs: 2g; Cholesterol: 195mg

Chicken Club Lettuce Wrap

If you've already got Salsa Shredded Chicken (page 131) prepped for the week, you can make any number of filling dinners in no time. This lettuce wrap is a great go-to meal when your only other option is the fast-food drive-through.

Prep time | **5 minutes**

NUT-FREE, EGG-FREE, UNDER 30 MINUTES

Serves 4

2 cups Salsa Shredded Chicken (page 131)

1 tomato, diced

1 avocado, sliced

6 Perfectly Cooked Bacon slices, (page 130), crumbled

4 tablespoons blue cheese crumbles

8 romaine lettuce leaves

Salt

Freshly ground black pepper

½ cup Dairy-Free Ranch Dressing (page 124)

1. To prepare the lettuce wraps, divide the chicken, tomato, avocado, bacon, and cheese evenly among the lettuce leaves. Season with salt and pepper.

2. Drizzle ranch dressing over each lettuce wrap and serve cold.

MAKE IT PALEO *Leave out the blue cheese and add an extra avocado to the filling.*

MACRONUTRIENTS **65% FAT**, 26% PROTEIN, 9% CARBS

PER SERVING Calories: 405; Total Fat: 29g; Saturated Fat: 7g; Protein: 26g; Total Carbs: 9g; Fiber: 4g; Net Carbs: 5g; Cholesterol: 76mg

Chicken-Broccoli Curry Bake

Growing up, I used to make a similar chicken curry dish with soup in a can. I am sure the carbs in that dish were out of control. This recipe shows how you can ketofy many of the high-carb recipes you enjoyed growing up. There is no reason you shouldn't be able to enjoy comfort food while living a ketogenic lifestyle; sometimes you just have to be a little bit creative.

Serves 8

Prep time | 10 minutes   *Cook time* | 30 minutes

NUT-FREE, EGG-FREE

Olive oil cooking spray

1 cup Mayonnaise (page 122)

1 cup sour cream

2 tablespoons freshly squeezed
   lemon juice

1 tablespoon curry powder

Salt

Freshly ground black pepper

3 cups shredded Colby-Jack
   cheese, divided

¼ cup shredded Parmesan cheese

3 cups cooked, shredded chicken
   breast (see page 12)

6 cups broccoli florets, blanched for
   2 minutes (see page 9),
   then drained

1. Preheat the oven to 375°F. Spray a 9-by-13-inch baking dish with the cooking spray.

2. In medium bowl, whisk together the mayonnaise, sour cream, lemon juice, and curry powder. Season with salt and pepper. Add 1½ cups of Colby-Jack cheese and the Parmesan cheese, and stir to combine.

3. Layer the shredded chicken and broccoli in the prepared baking dish. Top with the sour cream and cheese mixture, and gently stir it all together with a fork. Sprinkle the remaining 1½ cups of Colby-Jack cheese over the top of the casserole.

4. Bake for 30 to 35 minutes, or until the casserole is heated throughout and the cheese has browned on top.

5. Serve hot.

MACRONUTRIENTS **74% FAT**, 21% PROTEIN, 5% CARBS

PER SERVING Calories: 495; Total Fat: 41g; Saturated Fat: 15g; Protein: 26g; Total Carbs: 7g; Fiber: 2g; Net Carbs: 5g; Cholesterol: 95mg

Caprese-Stuffed Chicken

This keto-modified, Italian-inspired dish is super simple, and I love that it can be made in just one pan. The Caprese-Stuffed Chicken would be wonderful on a green salad with balsamic vinegar or over a bed of Creamed Spinach (page 85).

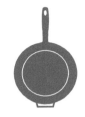

Prep time | 5 minutes *Cook time* | 20 minutes

NUT-FREE, EGG-FREE, UNDER 30 MINUTES

Serves 4

3 tablespoons olive oil, divided

4 skin-on, boneless chicken breasts

1 teaspoon garlic powder

Salt

Freshly ground black pepper

8 (1-ounce) slices mozzarella cheese

1 tomato, sliced

8 large basil leaves

1. Preheat the oven to 350°F.

2. Rub 1 tablespoon of olive oil on the chicken breasts, and season them with the garlic powder, salt, and pepper.

3. With a sharp knife, carefully cut each chicken breast horizontally in half, but do not cut all the way through the chicken breast. Create a pocket for layering the cheese, tomatoes, and basil.

4. Layer slices of mozzarella, tomatoes, and basil leaves in the middle of each chicken breast and close the pocket.

5. In a large cast iron skillet over medium heat, heat the remaining 2 tablespoons of olive oil. Place the chicken breasts in the skillet skin-side down. Cook for 4 to 5 minutes on each side, or until the skin is golden brown.

6. Transfer the skillet to the oven and bake for 8 to 12 minutes, or until the chicken is cooked through.

7. Serve immediately.

MAKE IT PALEO *Leave off the cheese and top the chicken with sliced avocado after cooking.*

MACRONUTRIENTS **66% FAT,** 32% PROTEIN, 2% CARBS

PER SERVING Calories: 465; Total Fat: 34g; Saturated Fat: 12g; Protein: 37g; Total Carbs: 3g; Fiber: 1g; Net Carbs: 2g; Cholesterol: 45mg

Chicken-Coconut Curry

This Indian-inspired dish is full of flavor and will lead your family to think you spent hours in the kitchen. Try serving this rich curry over Cauliflower Rice (see page 128) or spaghetti squash (see variation tip page 92), or add 4 cups of chicken broth to create a coconut-chicken curry soup. Coconut milk will enhance any dish and is a great alternative to heavy cream for those looking to limit dairy consumption.

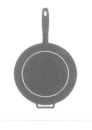

Serves 6

Prep time | 10 minutes   *Cook time* | 25 minutes

DAIRY-FREE, NUT-FREE, EGG-FREE, PALEO

2 tablespoons coconut oil

2 pounds boneless, skinless, chicken breasts, cut into ½-inch chunks

1 small yellow onion, diced

1 red bell pepper, chopped

2 tablespoons curry powder

Salt

Freshly ground black pepper

2 (15-ounce) cans full-fat coconut milk

Juice of 1 lime

2 cups thinly sliced red cabbage

1. In a large skillet over medium heat, melt the coconut oil. Add the cubed chicken, onion, and bell pepper, and season with curry powder, salt, and pepper. Sauté for 5 to 7 minutes, or until the vegetables have softened.

2. Add the coconut milk and lime juice to the mixture. Bring to a boil for 1 minute and reduce the heat to a simmer, cover, and simmer for 10 to 12 minutes, or until the chicken is cooked through and the sauce has thickened.

3. Add the sliced cabbage and cook for an additional 2 to 3 minutes, or until the cabbage has softened. Season with salt and pepper.

4. Serve hot in large bowls.

VARIATION TIP *Add ⅓ cup of chopped cashews to the mixture with the coconut milk and lime juice. You can also try folding in 6 ounces of fresh spinach instead of cabbage. Fold in spinach over medium heat and stir until spinach becomes wilted, 3 to 4 minutes.*

MACRONUTRIENTS **64% FAT**, 27% PROTEIN, 9% CARBS

PER SERVING Calories: 542; Total Fat: 39g; Saturated Fat: 30g; Protein: 37g; Total Carbs: 13g; Fiber: 2g; Net Carbs: 11g; Cholesterol: 87mg

Roasted Chicken and Vegetable Bake

This is the ultimate one-pan, quick-and-easy weeknight meal! I love sheet pan meals because they are so easy to switch up to keep things interesting. Get creative by substituting different proteins or low-carb veggies. Or add a few minced garlic cloves along with some diced bacon to the seasonings for a little extra oomph.

Serves 4

Prep time | 15 minutes   *Cook time* | 30 minutes

DAIRY-FREE, NUT-FREE, EGG-FREE, PALEO

Olive oil cooking spray
2 zucchini, chopped
1 head cauliflower, cut into florets
2 cups halved mushrooms
¼ cup olive oil or melted ghee
1 teaspoon garlic powder
Pinch salt
Pinch freshly ground black pepper
4 bone-in, skin-on chicken thighs

1. Preheat the oven to 375°F. Spray a sheet pan with the cooking spray.

2. In large, resealable plastic bag, combine the zucchini, cauliflower, and mushrooms with the olive oil, garlic powder, salt, and pepper.

3. Pat the chicken thighs dry with a paper towel, and add them to the plastic bag. Seal the bag and shake everything around to ensure that the chicken and vegetables are nicely coated with the oil and seasonings.

4. Empty the bag onto the prepared sheet pan, and arrange the chicken and vegetables in a single layer.

5. Bake for about 30 minutes, or until the chicken is crispy and the vegetables are browned.

6. Serve hot.

VARIATION TIP *Try adding broccoli, bell peppers, or cabbage to this easy sheet pan bake.*

MACRONUTRIENTS 58% FAT, 31% PROTEIN, 11% CARBS

PER SERVING Calories: 370; Total Fat: 24g; Saturated Fat: 5g; Protein: 29g; Total Carbs: 12g; Fiber: 5g; Net Carbs: 7g; Cholesterol: 89mg

Chicken-Stuffed Avocados

Avocados have a long list of health benefits, and they are a real keto superfood. They are low in carbs, high in healthy fats, and packed full of nutrients. What else could you ask for? One of the first questions I ask someone interested in trying keto is "How do you feel about avocados?" If they say they love them, they're in luck!

Serves 4

Prep time | 10 minutes   *Cook time* | 10 minutes

NUT-FREE, EGG-FREE, UNDER 30 MINUTES

2 avocados, halved

1 cup Salsa Shredded Chicken (page 131)

4 ounces cream cheese, at room temperature

1 tablespoon freshly squeezed lime juice

½ teaspoon ground cumin

½ teaspoon garlic powder

Salt

Freshly ground black pepper

1 cup shredded Colby-Jack cheese

1. Preheat the oven to 400°F. Line a sheet pan with parchment paper or aluminum foil.

2. Scoop the avocado flesh out of the shells into a medium bowl, being careful not to tear the shells. Set the shells aside. Add the chicken, cream cheese, lime juice, cumin, and garlic powder to the bowl, season with salt and pepper, and mix to combine.

3. Scoop the chicken mixture back into the avocado shells, and top with the shredded cheese.

4. Place the filled avocado shells on the prepared sheet pan, and bake until the cheese is melted, about 10 minutes.

5. Serve hot.

VARIATION TIP *Instead of shredded chicken, you could substitute tuna, salmon, or chopped hardboiled eggs.*

MACRONUTRIENTS **73% FAT**, 18% PROTEIN, 9% CARBS

PER SERVING Calories: 390; Total Fat: 32g; Saturated Fat: 12g; Protein: 18g; Total Carbs: 9g; Fiber: 6g; Net Carbs: 3g; Cholesterol: 80mg

Bunless Chicken-Bacon Burger

Keto means no sugar, no grains, which means you'll hear "bunless" quite often. What makes this lifestyle so maintainable is that you can stick to it even while traveling, going out with friends, or at business lunches and other events. Skipping the bread is a key habit to get into. This burger is so delicious, you won't miss the bun.

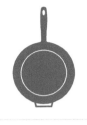

Serves 4

Prep time | 10 minutes   *Cook time* | 30 minutes

NUT-FREE

8 slices uncured bacon

4 (4-ounce) skin-on, boneless chicken breasts

Salt

Freshly ground black pepper

4 slices provolone or pepper Jack cheese

4 to 8 romaine lettuce leaves

¼ cup Mayonnaise (page 122)

1 avocado, sliced

1. Lay the bacon slices in a cold skillet. Set it over medium-low heat and cook until the bacon reaches your desired crispiness, about 8 minutes. Transfer the bacon from the skillet to a paper towel–lined plate.

2. Season the chicken breasts with salt and pepper, and place them in the skillet with the bacon grease over medium heat. Cook for 8 to 10 minutes on each side, or until the chicken is cooked all the way through.

3. Layer 2 pieces of bacon and 1 slice of cheese on each chicken breast. Divide the mayonnaise among 4 lettuce leaves, and place a chicken breast on each one. Top with the avocado slices, season with salt and pepper, and top with the remaining lettuce leaves.

4. Serve immediately.

MAKE IT PALEO *You can make this dish Paleo-friendly by leaving the cheese out and making the dairy-free version of Mayonnaise (page 122).*

MACRONUTRIENTS **64% FAT,** 31% PROTEIN, 5% CARBS

PER SERVING Calories: 435; Total Fat: 31g; Saturated Fat: 9g; Protein: 34g; Total Carbs: 5g; Fiber: 3g; Net Carbs: 2g; Cholesterol: 94mg

Roasted Cajun Chicken

This Cajun chicken is juicy and flavorful without a lot of complicated steps or ingredients. The trick to crispy, golden-brown chicken is making sure the thighs are patted dry, seasoned well, and cooked in a hot oven.

Prep time | 5 minutes   *Cook time* | 30 minutes

DAIRY-FREE, NUT-FREE, EGG-FREE, PALEO

Serves 4

4 tablespoons olive oil or melted ghee, plus more for preparing the pan

3 zucchini, chopped

1 bell pepper, seeded and diced

1 red onion, diced into 1-inch pieces

1 tablespoon Cajun seasoning

Salt

Freshly ground black pepper

4 (3½-ounce) bone-in, skin-on chicken thighs

1. Preheat the oven to 375°F. Grease a sheet pan with olive oil.

2. In large, resealable plastic bag, combine the zucchini, bell pepper, and onion with the olive oil or ghee and Cajun seasoning, and season with salt and pepper.

3. Pat the chicken thighs dry with paper towels and add them to the bag. Seal the bag and shake it up to ensure that the vegetables and meat are well-coated with the oil and seasonings.

4. Empty the bag onto the prepared sheet pan. Turn the thighs skin-side up and evenly arrange them on the sheet pan with the veggies.

5. Bake for about 30 minutes, or until the chicken is crispy and the vegetables are browned.

6. Serve hot.

VARIATION TIP *Replace the chicken with shrimp and bake at 400°F for 15 minutes. Add freshly squeezed lime juice after baking.*

MACRONUTRIENTS **61% FAT,** 28% PROTEIN, 11% CARBS

PER SERVING Calories: 340; Total Fat: 23g; Saturated Fat: 5g; Protein: 25g; Total Carbs: 10g; Fiber: 3g; Net Carbs: 7g; Cholesterol: 84mg

Chicken, Bacon, and Ranch Casserole

This is another casserole that might remind you of concoctions your mother used to make using cans of cream of chicken or cream of mushroom soup. This one is just as fast and easy to make, but much lower in carbs. You can save even more prep and cleanup time by mixing all of the ingredients together right in the baking dish instead of using a separate bowl.

Serves 6

Prep time | 10 minutes   *Cook time* | 20 minutes

NUT-FREE

Salted butter, for preparing the dish

4 cups Salsa Shredded Chicken (page 131)

10 slices Perfectly Cooked Bacon (page 130), crumbled

16 ounces frozen spinach, thawed and drained

2 garlic cloves, minced

1 cup Dairy-Free Ranch Dressing (page 124)

¼ cup sliced scallions, white and green parts (about 2 scallions)

1 cup shredded mozzarella cheese, divided

1 cup shredded Cheddar cheese, divided

1. Preheat the oven to 375°F. Grease a 9-by-13-inch baking dish with butter.

2. In a large bowl, combine the chicken, bacon, spinach, garlic, ranch dressing, scallions, ½ cup of mozzarella, and ½ cup of Cheddar. Mix until the ingredients are well incorporated. Pour into a greased 9-by-13-inch baking dish, and top with the remaining ½ cup each of mozzarella and Cheddar.

3. Bake for 15 to 20 minutes, or until the cheese turns golden brown and bubbly.

4. Serve hot.

MAKE IT PALEO *To make this dish Paleo, leave out the cheeses and top with sliced avocados before serving.*

MACRONUTRIENTS **64% FAT**, 31% PROTEIN, 5% CARBS

PER SERVING Calories: 521; Total Fat: 37g; Saturated Fat: 11g; Protein: 40g; Total Carbs: 7g; Fiber: 1g; Net Carbs: 6g; Cholesterol: 118mg

Parmesan-Crusted Chicken over Zucchini Noodles

Are you missing the crunch of breading or potato chips because of your low-carb lifestyle? Call me crazy, but pork rinds are an amazing alternative to them both! Pork rinds are very versatile, and here they provide the texture we all crave.

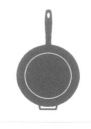

Serves 4

Prep time | 15 minutes   *Cook time* | 20 minutes

NUT-FREE, EGG-FREE

2 cups pork rinds, crushed

1 cup shredded Parmesan cheese

1 teaspoon garlic salt

Pinch salt

Pinch freshly ground black pepper

4 (4-ounce) boneless, skinless chicken breasts, pounded until flat

2 tablespoons coconut oil

1 cup Alfredo Sauce (page 126)

1 cup shredded mozzarella cheese

4 cups Zucchini Noodles (page 129)

1. Preheat the oven to 375°F.

2. In a large, resealable plastic bag, combine the pork rinds, Parmesan cheese, garlic salt, salt, and pepper, and shake to combine.

3. Add the chicken breasts, and shake to coat the chicken well with the pork rind mixture.

4. Heat a large cast iron skillet over medium heat. Add the coconut oil followed by the breaded chicken breasts. Cook for 3 to 4 minutes on each side, until the crust is golden brown.

5. Transfer the skillet to the oven and bake for 8 to 10 minutes, depending on thickness of your chicken breast. Remove the skillet from the oven and set the oven to broil.

6. Evenly distribute the alfredo sauce and mozzarella cheese over the chicken breasts. Broil until the cheese is melted and golden brown, 2 to 3 minutes.

7. Serve hot over the zucchini noodles.

MAKE AHEAD *Store uncooked, spiralized vegetable noodles refrigerated in an airtight container for up to 5 days.*

MACRONUTRIENTS **60% FAT**, 33% PROTEIN, 7% CARBS

PER SERVING Calories: 548; Total Fat: 36g; Saturated Fat: 19g; Protein: 46g; Total Carbs: 10g; Fiber: 2g; Net Carbs: 9g; Cholesterol: 145mg

Green Chile and Chicken Bake

This rich and creamy green chile and chicken bake is awesome served over Cheesy Cauliflower Rice (page 88), and pairs well with hot sauce, *pico de gallo*, guacamole, extra cheese, and sour cream. This will put all your Mexican food cravings to rest!

Prep time | 10 minutes   *Cook time* | 35 minutes

NUT-FREE, EGG-FREE

Serves 6

Salted butter, for preparing the baking dish

1 (8-ounce) package cream cheese, at room temperature

2 teaspoons garlic powder

2 teaspoons salt

1 teaspoon ground cumin

1 (4-ounce) can diced green chiles

6 (3½-ounce) skin-on, boneless chicken breasts

1 cup shredded Cheddar or Colby-Jack cheese

1. Preheat the oven to 375°F. Grease a 9-by-13-inch baking dish with butter.

2. In a medium bowl, mix the softened cream cheese, garlic powder, salt, and cumin until combined. Add the green chiles, and stir to incorporate.

3. Lay the chicken breasts in the prepared baking dish, and cover each one with the cream cheese mixture. Top each chicken breast with shredded cheese.

4. Bake for 30 to 35 minutes, or until the chicken is cooked through and the cheese is browned.

5. Serve hot.

MAKE AHEAD *This is another great recipe to double up on. You can serve one tonight and store the other in the freezer for a busy night in the future. Thaw the casserole in the refrigerator overnight and follow the baking instructions above when ready to cook.*

MACRONUTRIENTS **64% FAT, 33% PROTEIN, 3% CARBS**

PER SERVING Calories: 438; Total Fat: 31g; Saturated Fat: 14g; Protein: 37g; Total Carbs: 3g; Fiber: 0g; Net Carbs: 3g; Cholesterol: 149mg

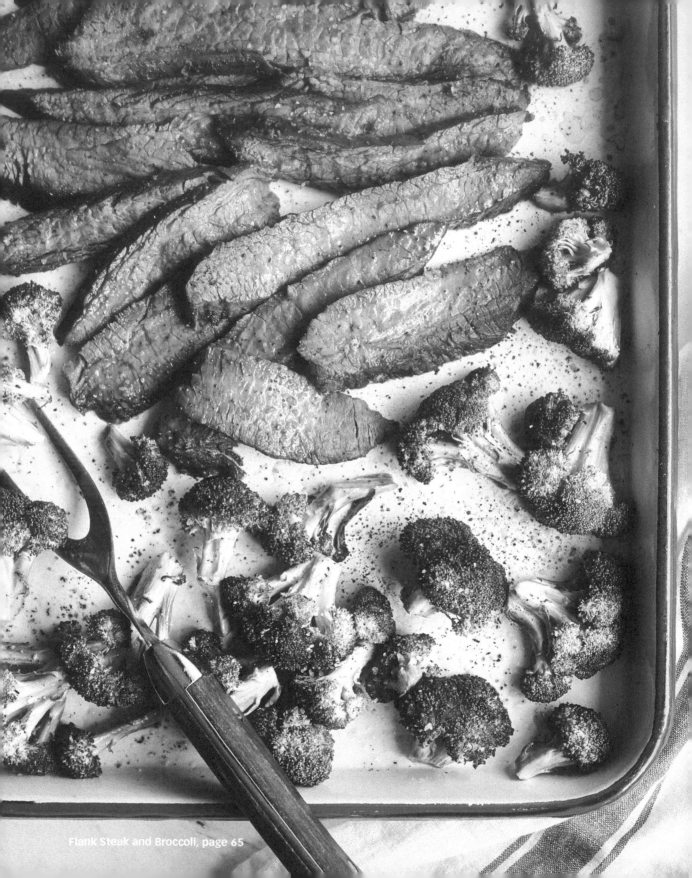

Flank Steak and Broccoli, page 65

CHAPTER 4

PORK
& BEEF

BLT Lettuce Wraps

You don't have to give up the delicious flavor of BLT sandwiches just because you've gone keto. This recipe delivers all of the flavors—the juicy tomatoes, creamy mayonnaise, salty bacon, and refreshingly crunchy lettuce—without the carbs.

Prep time | 10 minutes

DAIRY-FREE, NUT-FREE, PALEO, UNDER 30 MINUTES

Serves 2

2 tablespoons Mayonnaise (page 122) or your favorite low-carb or blue cheese dressing

8 large romaine lettuce leaves

Salt

Freshly ground black pepper

6 pieces Perfectly Cooked Bacon (page 130)

1 tomato, diced

1 avocado, chopped

Spoon the mayonnaise or dressing onto 4 of the lettuce leaves, and season with salt and pepper. Distribute the bacon, tomato, and avocado evenly among the 4 leaves. Top with the remaining lettuce leaves and serve immediately, 2 wraps per person.

VARIATION TIP *Add sliced hardboiled eggs and/or cheese to your wraps. These keto-friendly additions will add extra flavor and make these wraps even more filling.*

MACRONUTRIENTS **81% FAT,** 9% PROTEIN, 10% CARBS

PER SERVING Calories: 585; Total Fat: 54g; Saturated Fat: 15g; Protein: 13g; Total Carbs: 16g; Fiber: 8g; Net Carbs: 8g; Cholesterol: 61mg

Pork Carnitas Wraps

When you're trying to stick to a keto lifestyle, it's really help-ful to have back-up meal plans in place for those days when nothing goes as you expected. This easy pork dish is a great protein to have at the ready. Try using it as a topping for 5-Minute Chicharrones Nachos (page 58) or a garden salad, or stuff it into an avocado and top with Cheddar cheese, shredded cabbage, and freshly squeezed lime juice (my personal favorite).

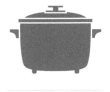

Serves 8

Prep time | 10 minutes   *Cook time* | 5 to 9 hours

NUT-FREE, EGG-FREE

1 tablespoon salt

2 teaspoons chili powder

2 teaspoons ground cumin

1 teaspoon freshly ground
   black pepper

1 teaspoon garlic powder

1 (3- to 5-pound) pork shoulder

Juice of 1 lime

FOR SERVING

Lettuce leaves

1 cup shredded sharp Cheddar cheese

½ cup sour cream

2 avocados, sliced

2 cups shredded cabbage

1 lime, cut into wedges

1. In a small bowl, stir together the salt, chili powder, cumin, pepper, and garlic powder. Rub the spice mixture all over the pork, and then place the pork in the slow cooker. Squeeze the lime juice over the top.

2. Cook on low for 8 hours or on high for 4 hours.

3. Transfer the meat to a platter and shred with two forks. It should fall apart easily. Return the shredded meat to the slow cooker with the juices, and cook on low for 30 to 60 minutes longer.

4. Wrap in lettuce leaves and top with cheese, sour cream, avocado, cabbage, and lime wedges.

MAKE IT PALEO *To make this dish Paleo, skip the cheese and sour cream when making your lettuce wraps.*

MACRONUTRIENTS **67% FAT,** 28% PROTEIN, 5% CARBS

PER SERVING Calories: 542; Total Fat: 41g; Saturated Fat: 15g; Protein: 36g; Total Carbs: 6g; Fiber: 4g; Net Carbs: 2g; Cholesterol: 140mg

Sloppy Joe Lettuce Wraps

Here is a modern, versatile, low-carb twist on a childhood favorite recipe. You may have noticed I use garlic powder or garlic salt frequently. If time isn't an issue, of course, fresh minced garlic is always better. If you have the time, use a clove of fresh, minced garlic instead. In dishes like this, where you sauté fresh garlic with the butter and onion, it really takes the dish up a level. This mixture is also great over low-carb noodles, like Zucchini Noodles (page 129).

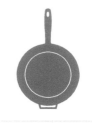

Serves 4

Prep time | 10 minutes   *Cook time* | 25 minutes

DAIRY-FREE, NUT-FREE, EGG-FREE, PALEO

1 tablespoon olive oil

1 green bell pepper, chopped

1 yellow onion, chopped

1 pound ground beef

½ cup sugar-free ketchup

1 teaspoon garlic powder

1 teaspoon prepared mustard

1 tablespoon Worcestershire sauce

1 tablespoon sugar substitute
   (such as Swerve)

Salt

Freshly ground black pepper

Romaine or iceberg lettuce leaves,
   for serving

1. In a large skillet over medium heat, heat the olive oil. Add the pepper and onion and cook, stirring frequently, until tender, 5 to 6 minutes. Add the ground beef and cook, stirring and breaking up the meat with a spatula, until it is browned and cooked through, 7 to 10 minutes more.

2. Stir in the ketchup, garlic powder, mustard, Worcestershire sauce, and sweetener, and season with salt and pepper. Bring to a boil, turn the heat down to low, and simmer for 10 minutes.

3. Serve hot in lettuce leaves.

VARIATION TIP *Try adding jalapeños, fresh zucchini, or sautéed cabbage to this dish. Don't be afraid to play with flavor profiles and get creative in your ketogenic lifestyle. As you become more familiar and comfortable with living this way, the possibilities in the kitchen and will continue to grow.*

MACRONUTRIENTS **58% FAT**, 35% PROTEIN, 7% CARBS

PER SERVING Calories: 272; Total Fat: 18g; Saturated Fat: 5g; Protein: 24g; Total Carbs: 5g; Fiber: 1g; Net Carbs: 4g; Cholesterol: 70mg

Bunless Bacon Cheeseburger

What's not to love in a bacon cheeseburger? This one won't disappoint. With seasoned beef patties, bacon, cheese, and all the fixings you expect on a burger, you won't miss the bun.

Prep time | 10 minutes   *Cook time* | 20 minutes

NUT-FREE

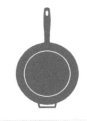

Serves 4

1 pound ground beef

Salt

Freshly ground black pepper

8 uncured bacon slices

8 slices American or Cheddar cheese

Iceberg lettuce

¼ cup Mayonnaise (page 122)

¼ cup sugar-free ketchup

2 tomatoes, sliced

1 avocado, sliced

1. Season the ground beef with salt and pepper, and form it into 4 patties.

2. In a large skillet over medium heat, cook the bacon until it reaches your desired crispiness, about 8 minutes. Transfer the bacon to a paper towel–lined plate and reserve. Remove and discard about half of the bacon grease, leaving enough in the pan to cook the burgers.

3. Return the skillet to the stovetop and cook the burgers over medium heat in the remaining bacon grease for about 5 minutes on each side, or until cooked to your desired doneness. When the patties are almost done cooking, place 2 pieces of cheese on each patty.

4. Transfer each cheeseburger to a bed of lettuce, and spread with the mayonnaise and ketchup. Top with the bacon, tomatoes, and avocados, and serve immediately.

VARIATION TIP *Try substituting ground pork for half of the ground beef when preparing your hamburger patties.*

MACRONUTRIENTS **66% FAT**, 26% PROTEIN, 8% CARBS

PER SERVING Calories: 560; Total Fat: 41g; Saturated Fat: 13g; Protein: 35g; Total Carbs: 11g; Fiber: 4g; Net Carbs: 7g; Cholesterol: 114mg

Bacon Cheeseburger Skillet

I use cast iron skillets more and more frequently in my kitchen. We are a busy family, and we try and keep the mess down during the work week, so being able to cook a whole meal in one pan keeps us on track with minimal cleanup. This Bacon Cheeseburger Skillet dinner is a perfect example, and for this recipe, any large skillet will do.

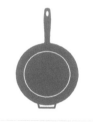

Serves 6

Prep time | 10 minutes   *Cook time* | 40 minutes

NUT-FREE, EGG-FREE

6 uncured bacon slices, diced

1 yellow onion, diced

1 pound ground beef

½ cup beef broth

2 cups cauliflower florets

¼ cup heavy (whipping) cream

1 cup shredded sharp Cheddar cheese

Salt

Freshly ground black pepper

1. In a large skillet over medium-high heat, cook the bacon until crisp, about 8 minutes. Transfer the bacon to a paper towel–lined plate.

2. Add the onion to the skillet with bacon grease and cook over medium-high heat, stirring frequently, until the onion becomes translucent, 3 to 5 minutes.

3. Reduce the heat to medium, and add the ground beef. Cook, stirring and breaking up the meat with a spatula, until the meat is browned, 7 to 10 minutes. Drain and discard some of the fat, leaving about 2 tablespoons of fat in the skillet.

4. Add the broth and cauliflower to the meat, cover, and cook for about 10 minutes, or until the cauliflower is tender. Remove the lid and simmer until the remaining liquid evaporates, 3 to 5 more minutes.

5. Add the cream and Cheddar, and mix until combined and melted. Season with salt and pepper and serve hot.

VARIATION TIP *This skillet meal leaves a lot of room to change things up. Try substituting ground bison, ground pork, or ground lamb for the ground beef and getting creative with cheese choices.*

MACRONUTRIENTS **61% FAT,** 32% PROTEIN, 7% CARBS

PER SERVING Calories: 284; Total Fat: 19g; Saturated Fat: 10g; Protein: 23g; Total Carbs: 5g; Fiber: 1g; Net Carbs: 4g; Cholesterol: 82mg

Taco Bar

It takes very little time to whip up a delicious skillet of taco meat filling, and it's a great thing to have in the refrigerator for busy weekdays. I use this seasoned meat for taco salads, Spanish omelets, and hearty soups and in recipes like the Vegetable Lasagna (page 84).

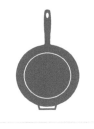

Serves 4

Prep time | 10 minutes   *Cook time* | 15 minutes

NUT-FREE, EGG-FREE, UNDER 30 MINUTES

1 pound ground beef

¼ cup taco seasoning

½ cup beef broth

TOPPINGS

½ cup shredded cabbage

½ cup shredded Monterey Jack cheese

¼ cup sour cream

1 tomato, diced

1 avocado, sliced

1 lime, cut into wedges

1. In a large skillet over medium heat, cook the beef until browned, 7 to 10 minutes. Add the taco seasoning and broth, and let simmer until the sauce thickens, about 5 minutes.

2. Serve immediately, garnished with the toppings.

MAKE AHEAD *I like to prep a double batch of this seasoned ground beef. After it cools completely, I divide it into single servings and put them in resealable plastic bags. The meat can be stored for up to 3 days in the refrigerator or in the freezer for up to 3 months.*

MACRONUTRIENTS **59% FAT,** 29% PROTEIN, 12% CARBS

PER SERVING Calories: 379; Total Fat: 24g; Saturated Fat: 10g; Protein: 28g; Total Carbs: 11g; Fiber: 4g; Net Carbs: 7g; Cholesterol: 89mg

5-Minute Chicharrones Nachos

Chicharrones, or pork rinds, may sound intimidating at first; at least they did to me. When I started my ketogenic journey, I found myself missing the crunch and saltiness of potato chips. I have found that pork rinds are a satisfying and low-carb but still crunchy and salty alternative. Here they're used in place of tortilla chips in a platter of nachos, complete with seasoned meat, melted cheese, avocado, sour cream, and jalapeño peppers. They're everything you expect from nachos, and still keto-friendly. You can find chicharrones in the chip aisle of your supermarket.

Serves 4

Prep time | 10 minutes *Cook time* | 5 minutes

NUT-FREE, EGG-FREE, UNDER 30 MINUTES

1 (16-ounce) bag chicharrones

½ pound cooked ground beef

2 cups shredded Cheddar or Monterey Jack cheese

1 (6-ounce) can black olives, drained and sliced

2 tomatoes, diced

1 avocado, sliced

½ cup sour cream

Jalapeño peppers, sliced, for serving

1. Set the oven to broil. Line a sheet pan with aluminum foil.

2. Spread the pork rinds out in a single layer on the prepared sheet pan. Top with the meat and cheese.

3. Broil until the cheese is melted, 3 to 5 minutes, watching carefully to prevent burning.

4. Serve the nachos immediately, topped with the olives, tomatoes, avocado, sour cream, and peppers.

MAKE AHEAD *Prepare the cooked meat ahead of time. Cook the beef in a large skillet over medium heat, stirring and breaking up the meat with a spatula, until browned, 7 to 10 minutes. Drain off the fat and let come to room temperature before storing, refrigerated in an airtight container, for up to 4 days, or in the freezer for up to 3 months.*

MACRONUTRIENTS **71% FAT,** 23% PROTEIN, 6% CARBS

PER SERVING Calories: 515; Total Fat: 41g; Saturated Fat: 19g; Protein: 30g; Total Carbs: 8g; Fiber: 3g; Net Carbs: 5g; Cholesterol: 98mg

Philly Cheesesteak Rollups

Philly cheesesteaks are something I ate far too frequently through my pregnancy. Where I went wrong was eating all the bread and fries. I ate them so often, it's crazy that Philly cheesesteaks are still a favorite. I promise you will not miss the bun, and this recipe will most likely become a staple in your kitchen.

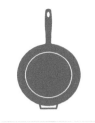

Serves 4

Prep time | 15 minutes *Cook time* | 20 minutes

NUT-FREE, EGG-FREE

1 pound sirloin tip steak

Salt

Freshly ground black pepper

¼ cup salted butter or ghee

1 green bell pepper, seeded and diced

1 yellow onion, diced

1 cup chopped mushrooms

6 slices provolone cheese

1. Pound the steak out to a thickness of about ¼ inch, and season it with salt and pepper.

2. In a large skillet over medium heat, melt the butter. Add the pepper, onion, and mushrooms and cook, stirring frequently, until tender, 5 to 6 minutes.

3. Spread the sautéed vegetables over the prepared steak in an even layer, and top with the cheese slices.

4. Starting with one of the short sides, roll the steak into a pinwheel, keeping the cheese tightly in the middle. Use toothpicks to secure the pinwheel every 2 inches, and then cut in between the toothpicks.

5. In the same skillet that you used to prepare the vegetables, cook the pinwheels over medium heat for 5 to 7 minutes on each side, until browned.

6. Serve warm, and remember to remove the toothpicks.

MAKE IT PALEO *Leave out the sliced cheese and add fresh spinach leaves instead.*

MACRONUTRIENTS **66% FAT**, 29% PROTEIN, 5% CARBS

PER SERVING Calories: 475; Total Fat: 35g; Saturated Fat: 19g; Protein: 33g; Total Carbs: 6g; Fiber: 1g; Net Carbs: 5g; Cholesterol: 127mg

German Brats and Sauerkraut

My mom lived in Austria during her twenties, so I've grown up with a love for German-influenced food. Each Christmas season, my mom hosts a magical German dinner with sauerkraut, brats, and schnitzel. The flavors in this dish always remind me of the holidays and the special memories shared around the table. Keep spicy mustard at the table for people to use as they like.

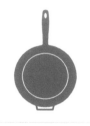

Serves 4

Prep time | 10 minutes   *Cook time* | 40 minutes

DAIRY-FREE, NUT-FREE, EGG-FREE, PALEO

¼ cup salted butter or ghee

½ yellow onion, chopped

½ head cabbage, thinly sliced

1 teaspoon garlic powder

Pinch salt

Pinch freshly ground black pepper

Juice of 1 lemon

1 cup sauerkraut, rinsed and drained

4 bratwursts or sweet Italian sausage links

Chopped fresh parsley, for garnish (optional)

1. Preheat the oven to 400°F.

2. In a large cast iron skillet or Dutch oven (with lid) over medium heat, melt the butter. Add the onion, cabbage, garlic powder, salt, and pepper. Cook, stirring frequently, until tender, 6 to 8 minutes.

3. Add the lemon juice and sauerkraut to the cabbage mixture, and toss until combined. Place the sausages on top of the sauerkraut, cover the pan, and transfer to the oven.

4. Bake for 20 minutes. Remove the lid and bake for 5 to 10 minutes more, until the sausages are cooked through.

5. Serve the sausages and the cabbage mixture hot, garnished with parsley (if using).

INGREDIENT TIP *When shopping for sauerkraut (and other fermented foods and beverages), look for products that contain live cultures. They deliver the good bacteria that make these foods so healthy.*

MACRONUTRIENTS **77% FAT**, 13% PROTEIN, 10% CARBS

PER SERVING Calories: 429; Total Fat: 37g; Saturated Fat: 16g; Protein: 14g; Total Carbs: 12g; Fiber: 4g; Net Carbs: 8g; Cholesterol: 94mg

Roasted Vegetables and Smoked Sausage

It doesn't get much simpler than this one-pan meal. Throw in any low-carb veggies you have on hand, and then dinner will be ready in no time. Sausage brings tons of flavor and makes it a filling and satisfying dish. In the unlikely event you have leftovers, throw them in your favorite broth (Bone Broth, page 121, is mine) and create an amazing smoked sausage soup.

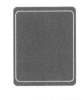

Serves 6

Prep time | 15 minutes   *Cook time* | 25 minutes

DAIRY-FREE, NUT-FREE, EGG-FREE, PALEO

2 cups chopped broccoli

1 green bell pepper, chopped

1 yellow onion, chopped

2 cups green beans, trimmed

1 pound smoked sausage, cut into
½-inch-thick slices

3 tablespoons olive oil or avocado oil

1 teaspoon salt

1 teaspoon freshly ground black pepper

½ teaspoon garlic powder

1. Preheat the oven to 425°F. Line a sheet pan with aluminum foil for easy cleanup.

2. Place the broccoli, bell pepper, onion, beans, and sausage in a single layer on the sheet pan. Drizzle the olive oil over the veggies and sausage, season with the salt, pepper, and garlic powder, and toss to make sure everything is evenly coated.

3. Bake for 25 minutes, or until the sausage is browned and the vegetables are tender. Halfway through the baking time, flip and stir the vegetables for best results.

4. Serve hot.

VARIATION TIP *Serve with Parmesan cheese, Dijon mustard, and fresh parsley.*

MACRONUTRIENTS **73% FAT,** 15% PROTEIN, 12% CARBS

PER SERVING Calories: 344; Total Fat: 28g; Saturated Fat: 10g; Protein: 13g; Total Carbs: 10g; Fiber: 3g; Net Carbs: 7g; Cholesterol: 51mg

Ribeye with Caramelized Onions and Mushrooms

There's nothing quite like a good, skillet-cooked ribeye to make you appreciate the keto diet. Topped with caramelized onion and mushrooms, this is one of my favorite meals. If you have any leftovers, pop them in a resealable plastic bag and refrigerate for up to 3 days. Slice the meat into thin strips (it's easiest to slice when it's cold), heat it up in a skillet, if you like, and then serve it over a Caesar salad or in an omelet with leftover sautéed onions and mushrooms and some Swiss cheese.

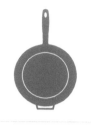

Serves 2

Prep time | **10 minutes, plus 5 minutes to rest**   *Cook time* | **15 minutes**

DAIRY-FREE, NUT-FREE, EGG-FREE, PALEO

2 (6-ounce) ribeye steaks

1 tablespoon olive oil

Salt

Freshly ground black pepper

2 tablespoons ghee or salted butter

1 yellow onion, sliced

1 cup sliced mushrooms

1. Pat the steaks dry with paper towels, then rub them with the olive oil. Season generously with salt and pepper.

2. In a large skillet over medium heat, heat the butter. Add the onion and cook, stirring frequently, for 3 to 5 minutes, until it starts to soften. Add the mushrooms and cook until the mushrooms are tender and the onion is translucent, another 5 minutes or so. Transfer the mixture to a paper towel–lined plate.

3. In the skillet over medium-high heat, grill the steak for 4 to 5 minutes on each side, to your desired doneness. Plate the steaks and let rest for 5 minutes.

4. Serve the steak immediately with the mushrooms and onion spooned over the top.

VARIATION TIP *To take this dish over the top, add Gorgonzola or blue cheese on top of the grilled mushrooms and onions. Place the skillet under the broiler until the cheese browns, being careful not to let it burn.*

MACRONUTRIENTS **54% FAT,** 41% PROTEIN, 5% CARBS

PER SERVING (with butter) Calories: 519; Total Fat: 31g; Saturated Fat: 12g; Protein: 52g; Total Carbs: 6g; Fiber: 1g; Net Carbs: 5g; Cholesterol: 161mg

Beef Stroganoff

For me, beef Stroganoff is the ultimate comfort food, and this keto-friendly version is no exception. Made with flavorful beef, butter, mushrooms, and sour cream, this dish will satisfy your cravings. In place of noodles, I like to serve this over Zucchini Noodles (page 129) or spaghetti squash (see variation tip page 92).

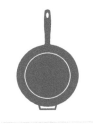

Serves 4

Prep time | 5 minutes   *Cook time* | 20 minutes

NUT-FREE, EGG-FREE, UNDER 30 MINUTES

1 pound ground beef

1 tablespoon salted butter

1 yellow onion, diced

2 cups mushrooms, sliced

2 garlic cloves, minced

1 cup beef broth

1 cup sour cream

¼ teaspoon xanthan gum

Salt

Freshly ground black pepper

Chopped fresh parsley, for garnish
  (optional)

Grated Parmesan cheese,
  for garnish (optional)

1. In a large skillet over medium-high heat, cook the ground beef, stirring and breaking it up with a spatula, until cooked through, 7 to 10 minutes. Drain the fat and transfer the meat to a paper towel–lined plate.

2. In the same skillet still over medium-high heat, melt the butter. Add the onion, mushrooms, and garlic and cook, stirring frequently, until the garlic is browned and the onion and mushrooms are tender, 5 to 7 minutes.

3. Add the broth, browned beef, sour cream, and xanthan gum to the skillet and cook, stirring, until the sauce is combined and thickened, 3 to 5 minutes.

4. Serve hot, garnished with the fresh parsley and grated Parmesan cheese (if using).

MAKE AHEAD *This recipe makes for great leftovers, freezes well, and can be paired with just about anything. After cooking, let it cool completely and store it in an airtight container in the refrigerator for 3 to 5 days or in the freezer for up to 3 months.*

MACRONUTRIENTS **61% FAT**, 30% PROTEIN, 9% CARBS

PER SERVING Calories: 369; Total Fat: 25g; Saturated Fat: 13g; Protein: 28g; Total Carbs: 8g; Fiber: 1g; Net Carbs: 7g; Cholesterol: 103mg

Meatloaf

My mind was blown when I discovered that you could form a meatloaf on a sheet pan rather than using a loaf pan. Baking meatloaf on an aluminum foil– or parchment-lined sheet pan makes for quick cleanup, leaving you more time to get creative with your meatloaf. Plus, you can add in any extra ingredients you happen to have and not worry about whether it will fit in the pan. You can make your loaves whatever size you like. Make a small one for a family of two, or a giant one for a get-together.

Serves 6

Prep time | **10 minutes, plus 10 minutes to rest**   *Cook time* | **40 minutes**

NUT-FREE

1 pound ground beef

1 pound ground pork

2 large eggs

1 cup pork rinds, crushed

½ cup grated Parmesan cheese

¼ cup heavy (whipping) cream

1 teaspoon prepared mustard

Salt

Freshly ground black pepper

¼ cup sugar-free ketchup or
   tomato paste

1 tablespoon apple cider vinegar

1 teaspoon sugar substitute
   (such as Swerve)

1. Preheat the oven to 400°F. Line a sheet pan with aluminum foil.

2. In large bowl, combine the beef, pork, eggs, pork rinds, cheese, cream, and mustard, and season with salt and pepper. Stir to mix well.

3. Form the mixture into a loaf shape on the prepared sheet pan.

4. In a small bowl, stir together the ketchup, vinegar, and sweetener. Brush the mixture on top of the formed loaf.

5. Bake for 35 to 40 minutes, or until nicely browned with an internal temperature of 160°F.

6. Remove from the oven and let rest for 5 to 10 minutes before slicing and serving.

MAKE AHEAD *Form the meatloaf mixture into 2 small loaves instead of 1 large loaf. Bake as directed, reducing the cooking time by about 10 minutes. Let cool to room temperature, wrap in aluminum foil, and freeze for up to 3 months.*

MACRONUTRIENTS **62% FAT,** 35% PROTEIN, 3% CARBS

PER SERVING Calories: 465; Total Fat: 32g; Saturated Fat: 13g; Protein: 41g; Total Carbs: 1g; Fiber: 0g; Net Carbs: 1g; Cholesterol: 203mg

Flank Steak and Broccoli

Flank steak is a fairly lean meat, so it can be tough. It cooks best at high heat for short periods, responds well to marinades, and is best sliced thinly across the grain (across the width). It's a great option when creativity and effort won't be happening before dinnertime, but you still want an enjoyable meal.

Serves 4

Prep time | 10 minutes, plus at least 30 minutes to marinate and 10 minutes to rest   *Cook time* | 10 minutes

DAIRY-FREE, NUT-FREE, EGG-FREE, PALEO

1 pound flank steak

6 tablespoons olive oil, divided

1 teaspoon garlic powder

1 teaspoon onion powder

Salt

Freshly ground black pepper

4 cups broccoli florets

1. In a large, resealable plastic bag, combine the steak and 3 tablespoons of olive oil with the garlic powder and onion powder. Season with salt and pepper. Refrigerate for at least 30 minutes, or up to 24 hours.

2. Set the oven broiler to high. Line a sheet pan with aluminum foil.

3. Place the steak and broccoli on the prepared sheet pan. Drizzle the remaining 3 tablespoons of olive oil over the broccoli, and season with salt and pepper. Toss until coated.

4. Cook under the broiler for 3 to 5 minutes, then flip the steak and continue to cook for 3 to 5 minutes more, or until the steak reaches your preferred doneness.

5. Let the steak rest for 10 minutes, then slice it thinly across the grain and serve with the roasted broccoli on the side.

VARIATION TIP *Switch this recipe up by using cauliflower florets, Brussels sprouts, and/or squash, which all roast well.*

MACRONUTRIENTS **69% FAT**, 26% PROTEIN, 5% CARBS

PER SERVING Calories: 380; Total Fat: 30g; Saturated Fat: 17g; Protein: 26g; Total Carbs: 5g; Fiber: 3g; Net Carbs: 2g; Cholesterol: 57mg

Barbecue Spare Ribs

Barbecue spare ribs are finger-licking good. The best part is that you just rub the spice mixture over them and pop them into the slow cooker. They can cook all day while you're at work, and when you come home, you get to enjoy scrumptious ribs for dinner. The Keto Coleslaw (page 73) complements these ribs well.

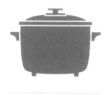

Serves 8

Prep time | 10 minutes   *Cook time* | 5 to 10 hours

DAIRY-FREE, NUT-FREE, EGG FREE, PALEO

2 pounds spare ribs

1 tablespoon salt

1 tablespoon garlic powder

1 tablespoon onion powder

1 tablespoon paprika

1 teaspoon ground cumin

1 teaspoon freshly ground
   black pepper

1. Pat the ribs dry with paper towels, and slice them into sections to fit in the slow cooker.

2. In a small bowl, stir together the salt, garlic powder, onion powder, paprika, cumin, and pepper. Rub the seasoning mixture all over the ribs.

3. Place the ribs in the slow cooker and cook on low for 8 to 10 hours or on high for 4 to 5 hours, until the meat is very tender and falling off the bones.

4. Serve hot.

MAKE AHEAD *This is a great make-ahead meal. You can even do the prep the night before. Just keep the seasoned ribs refrigerated overnight and let them come to room temperature before you put them in the slow cooker.*

MACRONUTRIENTS **65% FAT**, 34% PROTEIN, 1% CARBS

PER SERVING Calories: 263g; Total Fat: 19g; Saturated Fat: 7g; Protein: 21g; Total Carbs: 1g; Fiber: 0g; Net Carbs: 1g; Cholesterol: 78mg

Slow Cooker Pork Chili Colorado

This is a really easy dish to pop into a slow cooker in the morning and come home to a tasty, hot meal. Pork shoulder works particularly well in a slow cooker because the collagen softens with low, slow cooking and the fat content keeps it moist.

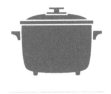

Serves 6

Prep time | 10 minutes   *Cook time* | 8 to 10 hours

EGG-FREE

2 pounds boneless pork shoulder, cut into 1-inch cubes

1 onion, chopped

2 tablespoons chili powder

1 tablespoon chipotle chili powder

1 teaspoon sea salt

Juice of 1 lime

1 avocado, cubed

½ cup grated Monterey Jack cheese

½ cup sour cream

¼ cup chopped, fresh cilantro

6 green onions, sliced

1. In a slow cooker, combine the pork shoulder, onion, chili powder, chipotle, and salt. Cover and cook on low for eight to ten hours, until the pork is soft.

2. Stir in the lime juice.

3. Serve garnished with the avocado, cheese, sour cream, cilantro, and onion.

TIP *If you can't find chipotle chili powder, buy whole dried chipotle chilies and grind them in a coffee or spice grinder.*

MACRONUTRIENTS **64% FAT**, 30% PROTEIN, 6% CARBS

PER SERVING Calories: 451; Total fat: 33g; Saturated fat: 12g; Protein: 32g; Total carbs: 7g; Fiber: 3g; Net Carbs: 4g; Cholesterol: 110mg

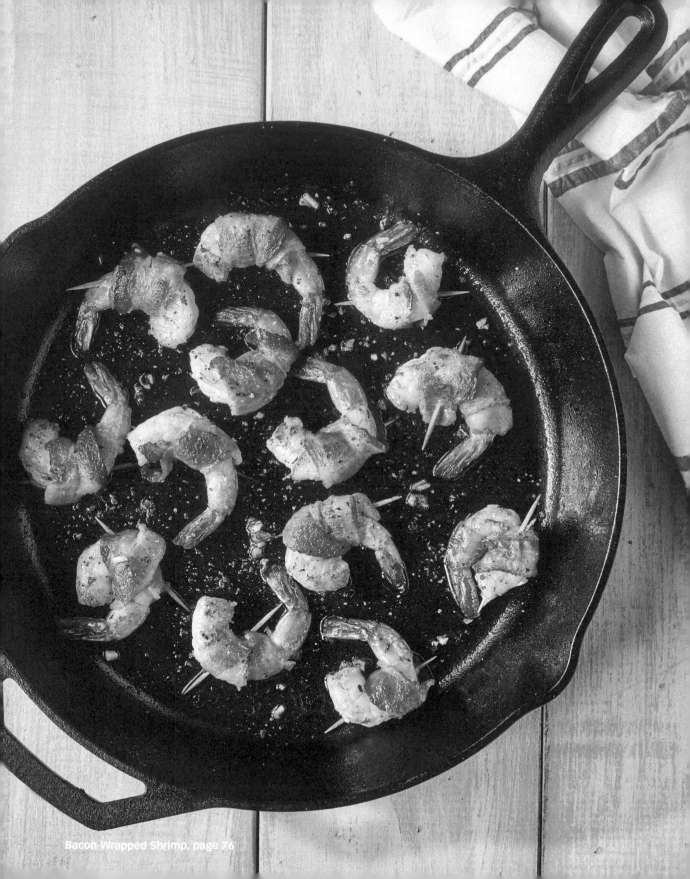

Bacon-Wrapped Shrimp, page 76

CHAPTER 5

FISH
& SEAFOOD

Tuna Salad Wraps

Tuna can be a real lifesaver when you are strapped for time on a crazy day. Tuna is not high in fat, so it's perfect for pairing with my homemade Mayonnaise (page 122) and avocado, which add all the fat you need to maintain your keto macro ratios.

Prep time | 15 minutes

NUT-FREE, PALEO, UNDER 30 MINUTES

Serves 2

2 (12-ounce) cans tuna, drained

½ red onion, diced

1 tomato, diced

1 tablespoon freshly squeezed lime juice

¼ cup Mayonnaise (page 122)

1 tablespoon prepared mustard

1 tablespoon celery seed

Salt

Freshly ground black pepper

1 avocado, sliced

Romaine lettuce leaves, for serving

1. In a large bowl, mix to combine the tuna, onion, tomato, lime juice, mayonnaise, mustard, and celery seed, and season with salt and pepper.

2. Serve with avocado, wrapped in romaine lettuce leaves.

VARIATION TIP *You can make this dish even more flavorful and satisfying by adding crumbled bacon and hardboiled eggs. And it doesn't have to be a wrap. Try serving the tuna salad with cucumber chips or pickles.*

MACRONUTRIENTS **64% FAT**, 26% PROTEIN, 10% CARBS

PER SERVING Calories: 506; Total Fat: 36g; Saturated Fat: 6g; Protein: 34g; Total Carbs: 13g; Fiber: 7g; Net Carbs: 6g; Cholesterol: 66mg

Crab-Stuffed Avocados

Crab meat is delicate, sweet, and delicious paired with melted butter, which makes it perfect for keto. You can enjoy crab alone or served in soups, sauces, and dips. Here it is paired with rich, creamy avocado, which is full of the healthy fats your body wants and needs.

Prep time | 15 minutes

Serves 4

DAIRY-FREE, NUT-FREE, PALEO, UNDER 30 MINUTES

2 avocados, halved

12 ounces crab meat

1 cup chopped celery

3 scallions, white and green parts, diced

6 tablespoons Mayonnaise (page 122)

Juice of 1 lemon

1 teaspoon paprika

Salt

Freshly ground black pepper

Lemon wedges, for garnish

1. Scoop the avocado meat out of the skin carefully, leaving a thin layer of meat attached to the skin. Dice the scooped-out avocado into small pieces, and place in a medium bowl.

2. Add the crab, celery, scallions, mayonnaise, lemon juice, and paprika, season with salt and pepper, and stir to combine.

3. Arrange an avocado shell cut-side up on each plate, and mound crab salad into each half. Serve immediately, garnished with lemon wedges.

INGREDIENT TIP *You might be tempted to substitute less expensive imitation crab for the crabmeat here, but watch out. Imitation crab contains 4 grams of carbohydrates per ounce!*

MACRONUTRIENTS **74% FAT**, 16% PROTEIN, 10% CARBS

PER SERVING Calories: 350; Total Fat: 29g; Saturated Fat: 4g; Protein: 14g; Total Carbs: 10g; Fiber: 7g; Net Carbs: 3g; Cholesterol: 81mg

One-Pan Salmon and Asparagus Bake

A good salmon fillet doesn't need much to turn it into a delicious meal. A little olive oil, salt, pepper, and freshly squeezed lemon juice go a long way. If your salmon fillets still have skin on them, cook them skin-side down. Salmon cooks quickly, so be careful not to overcook it.

Serves 4

Prep time | 15 minutes   *Cook time* | 10 minutes

DAIRY FREE, NUT-FREE, EGG FREE, PALEO, UNDER 30 MINUTES

4 (4- to 6-ounce) salmon fillets

5 tablespoons olive oil, divided

1 teaspoon garlic salt, divided

Juice of 1 lemon

1 pound asparagus, trimmed

Salt

Freshly ground black pepper

1. Set the oven to broil. Line a sheet pan with aluminum foil.

2. Rub each fillet with 2⅓ tablespoons of olive oil and ⅛ teaspoon of garlic salt. Arrange the fillets on the prepared sheet pan, and squeeze the lemon juice over the top.

3. Arrange the asparagus around the salmon, and drizzle it with remaining 2⅓ tablespoons of olive oil. Roll the asparagus around until coated, and season with salt and pepper.

4. Bake until the salmon is cooked through and flakes easily with a fork, 8 to 12 minutes.

5. Serve hot.

INGREDIENT TIP *When purchasing salmon, try to get the center cut. That's the best part of the fish for cooking because of its even thickness.*

MACRONUTRIENTS **65% FAT**, 31% PROTEIN, 4% CARBS

PER SERVING Calories: 475; Total Fat: 35g; Saturated Fat: 8g; Protein: 36g; Total Carbs: 6g; Fiber: 2g; Net Carbs: 4g; Cholesterol: 84mg

Baked Tilapia and Keto Coleslaw

We love the crunch and tang of this coleslaw at our house. It pairs perfectly with the lemon-pepper tilapia and avocado (what doesn't pair well with avocados though?). If you are making this for fewer than four people, keep the dressing separate from the cabbage until you eat the leftovers. The crunch of the cabbage is the best part!

Serves 4

Prep time | 15 minutes   *Cook time* | 15 minutes

DAIRY-FREE, NUT-FREE, PALEO, UNDER 30 MINUTES

FOR THE FISH

Olive oil cooking spray (optional)
4 (4- to 6-ounce) tilapia fillets
2 tablespoons olive oil or avocado oil
2 teaspoons lemon-pepper seasoning

FOR THE COLESLAW

½ cup Mayonnaise (page 122)
2 tablespoons freshly squeezed
  lemon juice
1 tablespoon prepared mustard
1 tablespoon apple cider vinegar
1 tablespoon sugar substitute
  (such as Swerve)
1 teaspoon celery seeds
Salt
Freshly ground black pepper
1 head cabbage, sliced

FOR SERVING

1 avocado, sliced
1 lemon, sliced

TO MAKE THE FISH

1. Preheat the oven to 425°F. Line a sheet pan with aluminum foil or spray with cooking spray.

2. Rub the fish fillets with the olive oil, and season with lemon pepper.

3. Arrange the fish in a single layer on the sheet pan and bake for about 15 minutes, or until the fish is white, opaque, and cooked through.

TO MAKE THE COLESLAW

1. While the fish is baking, make the dressing for the coleslaw. In a small bowl, whisk together the mayonnaise, lemon juice, mustard, vinegar, sugar substitute, and celery seeds, and season with salt and pepper.

2. When the fish is finished baking, let it rest on the cutting board for 5 to 10 minutes.

3. Divide the cabbage and avocado evenly among 4 bowls. Add the dressing, top each serving with a fish fillet, garnish with a lemon slice, and serve.

Continued

Baked Tilapia and Keto Coleslaw *Continued*

INGREDIENT TIP *I know that when you're trying to get a meal on the table on a busy weeknight, every second counts. You can buy presliced cabbage for coleslaw to save time on prep.*

MACRONUTRIENTS **64% FAT,** 21% PROTEIN, 15% CARBS

PER SERVING Calories: 495; Total Fat: 36g; Saturated Fat: 6g; Protein: 28g; Total Carbs: 19g; Fiber: 10g; Net Carbs: 9g; Cholesterol: 33mg

Lemon Cream Tilapia Bake

This simple fish dish is always a hit with my family. Since I'm usually cooking for just my husband, toddler, and myself, I make the whole recipe so that we'll have leftovers. Add some sliced avocado and my favorite low-carb salad dressing, and that's two dinners covered.

Serves 4

Prep time | 10 minutes *Cook time* | 15 minutes

NUT-FREE, EGG-FREE, UNDER 30 MINUTES

4 (4- to 6-ounce) tilapia fillets (you can substitute halibut or another white fish)

1 teaspoon garlic powder

Salt

Freshly ground black pepper

¼ cup (½ stick) salted butter, at room temperature

¼ cup heavy (whipping) cream

¼ cup cream cheese, at room temperature

1 tablespoon prepared mustard

2 tablespoons freshly squeezed lemon juice

1. Preheat the oven to 400°F.

2. In a 9-by-13-inch baking dish, arrange the fillets in a single layer. Season with garlic powder, salt, and pepper.

3. In a small bowl, mix to combine the butter, cream, cream cheese, mustard, and lemon juice. Microwave in 30 second intervals, stirring in between, until the mixture is smooth, 1 to 2 minutes total.

4. Pour the sauce over the top of the fish and bake for 10 to 15 minutes, or until the fish is white, opaque, and cooked through.

5. Serve immediately.

INGREDIENT TIP *If you forgot to take the frozen fish out of the freezer, don't fret! Put the frozen fish in a resealable plastic bag to protect it. Put the bag in a large bowl in the sink and run cool water over the fish until it is thawed.*

MACRONUTRIENTS 59% FAT, 38% PROTEIN, 3% CARBS

PER SERVING Calories: 369g; Total Fat: 25g; Saturated Fat: 15g; Protein: 35g; Total Carbs: 2g; Fiber: 0g; Net Carbs: 2g; Cholesterol: 150mg

Bacon-Wrapped Shrimp

For this dish, plump shrimp are wrapped in flavorful bacon and then cooked in a skillet until crisp. The combination of the juicy shrimp and crispy, salty bacon is divine. If you like your bacon extra crispy, I recommend partially cooking it before wrapping the shrimp. This will guarantee a delectably crunchy bacon-wrapped shrimp.

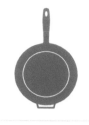

Serves 4

Prep time | 15 minutes   *Cook time* | 10 minutes

DAIRY-FREE, NUT-FREE, EGG-FREE, PALEO, UNDER 30 MINUTES

⅓ cup olive oil

1 teaspoon lemon zest

Juice of 1 lemon

4 garlic cloves, minced

24 large shrimp, peeled and deveined

12 uncured bacon slices,
   halved crosswise

Salt

Freshly ground black pepper

1. In a small bowl, mix to combine the olive oil, lemon zest, lemon juice, and garlic.

2. Wrap each shrimp with bacon, using a toothpick to secure. Brush the shrimp with the olive oil mixture, and season with salt and pepper.

3. Heat a large skillet over medium-high heat and cook each shrimp, turning occasionally, until the bacon is browned and crisp on all sides and the shrimp are pink, opaque, and cooked through, 5 to 6 minutes.

4. Serve hot.

ALLERGEN TIP *If you're cooking for someone with a shellfish allergy, substitute chicken strips for the shrimp.*

MACRONUTRIENTS **78% FAT,** 21% PROTEIN, 1% CARBS

PER SERVING Calories: 287; Total Fat: 25g; Saturated Fat: 6g; Protein: 16g; Total Carbs: 2g; Fiber: 0g; Net Carbs: 2g; Cholesterol: 130mg

Shrimp Alfredo with Zucchini Noodles

It doesn't get more keto than this! Zucchini noodles are an awesome alternative to regular high-carb noodles, and they won't leave you feeling bloated like a big bowl of pasta can, either. If you don't have a spiralizer, use a potato peeler or sharp knife to cut the zucchini into thin strips.

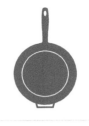

Serves 3

Prep time | 10 minutes   *Cook time* | 15 minutes

NUT-FREE, EGG-FREE, UNDER 30 MINUTES

3 tablespoons salted butter, divided

1 pound large shrimp, peeled and deveined

½ teaspoon sea salt

½ teaspoon freshly ground black pepper

4 zucchini, spiralized

1½ cups Alfredo Sauce (page 126)

¼ cup grated Parmesan cheese

1. In a large skillet over medium heat, melt 1 tablespoon of butter. Add the prepared shrimp, and season with salt and pepper.

2. Cook the shrimp, stirring occasionally, for 4 to 6 minutes, or until the shrimp are pink, opaque, and cooked through. Transfer the shrimp to a paper towel–lined plate.

3. In the skillet, melt the remaining 2 tablespoons of butter. Add the zucchini noodles and toss until coated with butter. Sauté for 3 to 5 minutes, or until the noodles reach your desired texture.

4. Add the Alfredo sauce and shrimp and heat until warm, 3 to 5 minutes.

5. Serve immediately in bowls topped with Parmesan cheese.

VARIATION TIP *Add flavor and texture to this dish with cooked and crumbled bacon or sautéed mushrooms.*

MACRONUTRIENTS **60% FAT**, 28% PROTEIN, 12% CARBS

PER SERVING Calories: 558; Total Fat: 37g; Saturated Fat: 16g; Protein: 39g; Total Carbs: 17g; Fiber: 3g; Net Carbs: 14g; Cholesterol: 327mg

Sheet Pan Shrimp Fajitas

Making fajitas for a quick-and-easy weeknight meal is always a good idea. This recipe is super simple and satisfies any Mexican food craving—without the beans and rice. Fajitas are a great option when eating out, too. Just ask the server to hold the starches and enjoy the guacamole, sour cream, and cheese!

Serves 4

Prep time | 10 minutes   *Cook time* | 10 minutes

NUT-FREE, EGG-FREE, UNDER 30 MINUTES

Olive oil cooking spray (optional)

2 pounds large shrimp, peeled and deveined

1 green bell pepper, seeded and chopped

1 red bell pepper, seeded and chopped

1 red onion, chopped

¼ cup plus 1 tablespoon olive oil or avocado oil

1 teaspoon salt

1 teaspoon freshly ground black pepper

1 teaspoon garlic powder

1 teaspoon ground cumin

Juice of 1 lime

1 avocado, sliced

½ cup sour cream

1 cup shredded Colby-Jack cheese

1. Preheat the oven to 400°F. Line a sheet pan with aluminum foil or spray with cooking spray.

2. In a large, resealable plastic bag, combine the shrimp, bell peppers, onion, olive oil, salt, pepper, garlic powder, cumin, and lime juice, and shake until everything is evenly coated with oil and seasonings.

3. Pour the shrimp mixture onto the prepared sheet pan and bake for about 10 minutes, or until the shrimp are pink, opaque, and cooked through.

4. Serve hot topped with the avocado slices, sour cream, and shredded cheese.

MACRONUTRIENTS **58% FAT,** 34% PROTEIN, 8% CARBS

PER SERVING Calories: 635; Total Fat: 41g; Saturated Fat: 12g; Protein: 54g; Total Carbs: 14g; Fiber: 4g; Net Carbs: 10g; Cholesterol: 380mg

Crab Cakes

When working with crabmeat, fresh is best. Try to find large lump crabmeat. When incorporating crabmeat into your dish, fold it in gently during the final step of prep, and avoid overmixing. Crab cakes are great served with a fried egg and avocado or Hollandaise Sauce (page 125).

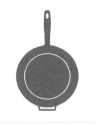

Serves 4

Prep time | 10 minutes   *Cook time* | 10 minutes

DAIRY-FREE, NUT-FREE, PALEO, UNDER 30 MINUTES

1 large egg

1 tablespoon freshly squeezed lemon juice

1 teaspoon prepared mustard

3 tablespoons Mayonnaise (page 122)

1 pound lump crabmeat

3 tablespoons coconut flour

Salt

Freshly ground black pepper

¼ cup coconut oil

1. In small bowl, whisk together the egg, lemon juice, mustard, and mayonnaise. Gently fold in the crabmeat, being careful not to break the crab up. Add the coconut flour, season with salt and pepper, and stir gently to combine.

2. Form the crab mixture into 6 patties.

3. In a large skillet over medium heat, melt the coconut oil. Cook the crab cakes for 3 to 5 minutes on each side.

4. Serve immediately.

VARIATION TIP *For a little more heft and crunch, add ⅔ cup of crushed pork rinds to the crab cake mixture before cooking.*

MACRONUTRIENTS **61% FAT**, 31% PROTEIN, 8% CARBS

PER SERVING (2 patties) Calories: 498; Total Fat: 34g; Saturated Fat: 19g; Protein: 38g; Total Carbs: 10g; Fiber: 5g; Net Carbs: 5g; Cholesterol: 197mg

Creamy Seafood Casserole

Keto makes casseroles a lot more fun and completely guilt-free. As with most casseroles, you can prepare this one ahead of time, cover, and freeze or refrigerate for a convenient weeknight meal that everyone will love. Whenever you want to add an extra kick to your casseroles, spread crushed pork rinds over the top before baking.

Serves 6

Prep time | 10 minutes   *Cook time* | 30 minutes

NUT-FREE, EGG-FREE

Olive oil cooking spray

1¼ cup heavy (whipping) cream or full-fat coconut milk

2 tablespoons salted butter

¼ cup shredded sharp Cheddar cheese

½ cup shredded Swiss cheese

¼ cup grated Parmesan cheese

2 teaspoons Worcestershire sauce

¼ teaspoon paprika

¼ teaspoon ground nutmeg

Salt

Freshly ground black pepper

1 pound white fish, cut into bite-sized pieces

½ pound large shrimp, peeled and deveined

1. Preheat the oven to 350°F. Spray a 9-by-13-inch baking dish with cooking spray.

2. In a large microwave-safe bowl, combine the cream, butter, cheeses, Worcestershire sauce, paprika, and nutmeg, and season with salt and pepper. Microwave in 30-second intervals, stirring in between, until the cheese is melted and the mixture is smooth.

3. Place the seafood in the prepared baking dish, pour the sauce over the top, and season with additional salt and pepper.

4. Bake for 20 minutes, or until the sauce becomes bubbly and the fish is opaque and cooked through.

5. Serve hot.

VARIATION TIP *If you're looking for a way to add a green vegetable to this meal, stir 2 cups of broccoli florets into the mixture before baking.*

MACRONUTRIENTS **64% FAT,** 33% PROTEIN, 3% CARBS

PER SERVING Calories: 391; Total Fat: 28g; Saturated Fat: 17g; Protein: 31g; Total Carbs: 3g; Fiber: 0g; Net Carbs: 3g; Cholesterol: 220mg

Pan-Seared Scallops with Lemon Beurre Blanc

Beurre blanc is a fancy name for white butter sauce, and when it's drizzled over scallops and sautéed spinach, it adds rich flavor.

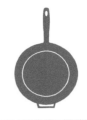

Prep time | 10 minutes   *Cook time* | 15 minutes

NUT-FREE, EGG-FREE, UNDER 30 MINUTES

Serves 2

10 tablespoons unsalted butter, divided

3 cups baby spinach

1 teaspoon sea salt, divided

¼ teaspoon freshly cracked black pepper, divided

10 sea scallops, rinsed and patted dry

2 tablespoons minced shallot

½ cup dry white wine, such as Chardonnay

Zest and juice of ½ lemon

2 tablespoons chopped basil

1. Cut 6 tablespoons of butter into ½-inch pieces and place them in the freezer so they get very cold while you work.

2. In a large skillet, heat 2 tablespoons of butter on medium-high until it bubbles. Add the spinach, ½ teaspoon of salt, and ⅛ teaspoon of pepper and cook, stirring for a minute or two, until the spinach wilts. Set aside on a platter tented with foil to keep warm.

3. Wipe out the skillet with a paper towel to remove any moisture left from the spinach. Season the scallops with the remaining ½ teaspoon of sea salt and ⅛ teaspoon of pepper. Heat the remaining two tablespoons of butter in the pan on medium-high heat until it bubbles. Add the scallops and cook, two to three minutes per side, until they are seared on both sides. Remove the scallops from the pan with tongs and set aside on the platter with the spinach, tented with foil to keep warm.

4. Add the shallot, wine, lemon juice, and lemon zest to the pan. Bring to a simmer and reduce the heat to medium-low. Simmer until the liquid is reduced by half, about five minutes.

5. Remove the butter from the freezer and whisk the very cold butter into the sauce, 1 piece at a time until it is all incorporated.

6. Place the scallops on the spinach and drizzle the beurre blanc over the top. Garnish with the basil.

MACRONUTRIENTS **80% FAT**, 10% PROTEIN, 10% CARBS

PER SERVING: Calories: 634; Total fat: 58g; Saturated fat: 36g; Protein: 15g; Total carbs: 7g; Fiber: 1g; Net carbs: 6g; Cholesterol: 175mg

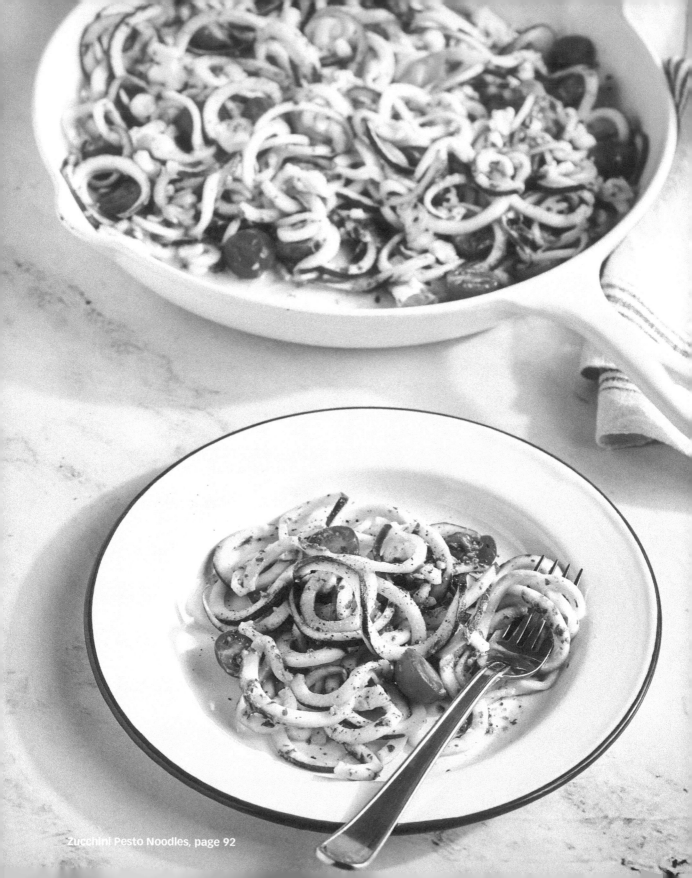

Zucchini Pesto Noodles, page 92

CHAPTER
6

VEGETABLE MAINS

Vegetable Lasagna

This is a classic dish with a keto twist. Zucchini cut into the shape of lasagna noodles works a healthy vegetable into the dish and stands in for high-carb noodles. Serve this lasagna with a vegetable-filled green salad, and you have a satisfying meal that's appropriate for just about any occasion.

Serves 6

Prep time | 15 minutes, plus 10 minutes to rest   *Cook time* | 30 minutes

NUT-FREE, VEGETARIAN

2 tablespoons salted butter, for preparing the baking dish

2 cups ricotta cheese

1½ cups grated Parmesan cheese

2 large eggs

Salt

Freshly ground black pepper

1 cup low-carb marinara sauce

4 large zucchini, sliced lengthwise into thin sheets

2 cups shredded mozzarella cheese

1. Preheat the oven to 350°F. Grease a 9-by-13-inch baking dish with the butter.

2. In a medium bowl, stir together the ricotta cheese, Parmesan cheese, and eggs, and season with salt and pepper.

3. Spread a bit of the marina sauce in the bottom of the prepared baking dish. Cover the sauce with a layer of zucchini strips. Top with about one-third of the remaining marinara sauce, one-third of the ricotta mixture, and one-third of the mozzarella. Repeat two more times, until all ingredients are used up, ending with a layer of mozzarella. Season with salt and pepper.

4. Bake for about 30 minutes, or until the cheese is melted and the zucchini is tender.

5. Let rest for 10 minutes before slicing and serving.

MACRONUTRIENTS **61% FAT,** 29% PROTEIN, 10% CARBS

PER SERVING Calories: 464; Total Fat: 31g; Saturated Fat: 19g; Protein: 34g; Total Carbs: 12g; Fiber: 2g; Net Carbs: 10g; Cholesterol: 154mg

Creamed Spinach

Keto generously brings back the flavorful ingredients that we tended to eat sparingly in the past. This dish is a perfect example. Healthy spinach is cooked with rich cream, cream cheese, sour cream, butter, and Parmesan cheese for an extremely tasty dish. If you've always liked spinach, you will love this upgrade. If you never quite understood Popeye's passion, this version may just convince you to add this nutrient-rich vegetable to your list of favorites.

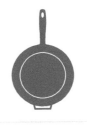

Serves 4

Prep time | 5 minutes   *Cook time* | 10 minutes

NUT-FREE, EGG-FREE, VEGETARIAN, UNDER 30 MINUTES

4 tablespoons salted butter, divided

2 garlic cloves, minced

2 (10-ounce) packages frozen chopped spinach, thawed and drained

4 ounces cream cheese

2 tablespoons sour cream

½ cup heavy (whipping) cream

½ cup grated Parmesan cheese

Pinch salt

Pinch freshly ground black pepper

1. In a large skillet over medium heat, melt 2 tablespoons of butter. Cook the garlic until it is browned, 1 to 2 minutes. Stir in the spinach and cook until any liquid that is released evaporates, about 5 minutes.

2. Add the cream cheese, sour cream, heavy cream, Parmesan cheese, salt, pepper, and the remaining 2 tablespoons of butter. Cook, stirring, until the butter and cream cheese are melted, about 3 minutes. Serve hot.

INGREDIENT TIP *You can use fresh spinach, but it will take about 20 cups of fresh spinach to get the same amount as the frozen spinach listed in the recipe.*

MACRONUTRIENTS **84% FAT**, 10% PROTEIN, 6% CARBS

PER SERVING Calories: 387; Total Fat: 37g; Saturated Fat: 22g; Protein: 10g; Total Carbs: 6g; Fiber: 2g; Net Carbs: 4g; Cholesterol: 116mg

Roasted Cauliflower and Broccoli

I am obsessed with broccoli and cauliflower, and after trying this recipe, I'm pretty sure you'll be in the same boat. You can switch this recipe up with freshly squeezed lemon juice, sliced almonds, or your favorite keto-friendly cheese sauce on top.

Serves 4

Prep time | 10 minutes   *Cook time* | 20 minutes

NUT-FREE, EGG-FREE, VEGETARIAN

---

2 cups cauliflower florets

2 cups broccoli florets

¼ cup olive oil or avocado oil

⅔ cup grated Parmesan cheese

1 teaspoon garlic powder

1 teaspoon onion powder

1 teaspoon salt

½ teaspoon freshly ground
  black pepper

1. Preheat the oven to 400°F. Line a sheet pan with aluminum foil.

2. In a large, resealable plastic bag or large bowl, toss the cauliflower, broccoli, and olive oil with about half of the Parmesan cheese and the garlic powder, onion powder, salt, and pepper until the vegetables are evenly coated.

3. Arrange the vegetables on the prepared sheet pan, making sure they aren't too crowded.

4. Bake for 15 to 20 minutes, turning the ingredients halfway through cooking, until the edges are browned.

5. Sprinkle the remaining Parmesan cheese over the top, season with additional salt and pepper if desired, and serve immediately.

MAKE IT PALEO *To make this dish paleo, leave out the Parmesan cheese and enjoy!*

MACRONUTRIENTS **76% FAT**, 15% PROTEIN, 9% CARBS

PER SERVING Calories: 221; Total Fat: 19g; Saturated Fat: 5g; Protein: 9g; Total Carbs: 5g; Fiber: 3g; Net Carbs: 2g; Cholesterol: 13mg

Brussels Sprouts with Bacon

This recipe is for all those people who cringe when they hear "Brussels sprouts." I was in the same boat—I hated their smell and thought they were always mushy. But I promise, these oven-roasted Brussels sprouts with bacon and healthy fat will turn your perspective around.

Serves 4

Prep time | 10 minutes   *Cook time* | 30 minutes

DAIRY-FREE, NUT-FREE, EGG-FREE, PALEO

Olive oil cooking spray (optional)

4 cups Brussels sprouts, trimmed and halved

¼ cup olive oil or avocado oil

2 teaspoons garlic salt

12 uncured bacon slices, cut into 1-inch pieces

1. Preheat the oven to 400°F. Line a sheet pan with aluminum foil or spray with cooking spray.

2. In a large resealable plastic bag or a large bowl, combine the Brussels sprouts, olive oil, garlic salt, and bacon, and toss to mix well.

3. Spread the mixture evenly onto the prepared sheet pan.

4. Roast for 20 to 30 minutes, stirring once during cooking, until the Brussels sprouts are tender and the bacon is cooked through.

5. Serve hot.

VARIATION TIP *For extra flavor, stir a dash of balsamic vinegar and grilled onions into the dish after baking.*

MACRONUTRIENTS **85% FAT,** 9% PROTEIN, 6% CARBS

PER SERVING Calories: 512; Total Fat: 49g; Saturated Fat: 14g; Protein: 12g; Total Carbs: 9g; Fiber: 3g; Net Carbs: 6g; Cholesterol: 54mg

Cheesy Cauliflower Rice

Remember the days of the loaded potatoes we loved, before the guilt era set in? Here's the keto twist: Use riced cauliflower, more vegetables, and less carbs, all while maintaining amazing flavors. The Cauliflower Rice recipe (page 128) provides an ideal background for building your own.

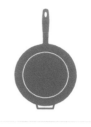

Serves 4

Prep time | 10 minutes   *Cook time* | 15 minutes

NUT-FREE, EGG-FREE, VEGETARIAN, UNDER 30 MINUTES

3 tablespoons salted butter

1 yellow onion, diced

4 cups Cauliflower Rice (page 128)

¹⁄₃ cup heavy (whipping) cream

1 cup shredded Cheddar cheese

1 teaspoon garlic powder

1 teaspoon onion powder

Salt

Freshly ground black pepper

1. In a large skillet over medium heat, melt the butter. Add the onion and cook, stirring frequently, until translucent, 3 to 5 minutes. Add the cauliflower rice and continue to cook for an additional 5 minutes, stirring often.

2. Stir in the cream, cheese, garlic powder, and onion powder, and season with salt and pepper. Cook until the cheese is melted, 3 to 5 minutes.

3. Serve hot.

INGREDIENT TIP *You can buy "riced cauliflower," or cauliflower that has been finely chopped to the sizes and shape of rice, either frozen or in the produce section. This product will save you a lot of time and hassle.*

MACRONUTRIENTS **76% FAT**, 13% PROTEIN, 11% CARBS

PER SERVING Calories: 297; Total Fat: 25g; Saturated Fat: 16g; Protein: 10g; Total Carbs: 10g; Fiber: 3g; Net Carbs: 7g; Cholesterol: 79mg

Cheese-Stuffed Zucchini Boats

Zucchini makes a great vehicle for filling with just about anything you like—as long as it is low-carb. Here they're stuffed with a rich and flavorful mix of cheeses and spinach.

Prep time | 15 minutes   *Cook time* | 30 minutes

NUT-FREE, EGG-FREE, VEGETARIAN

Serves 6

4 large zucchini

1½ cups ricotta cheese

2 cups shredded mozzarella cheese, divided

½ cup Parmesan cheese, grated

1 (10-ounce) package frozen spinach, thawed and drained

Salt

Freshly ground black pepper

1½ cups low-carb marinara sauce

4 fresh basil leaves, chopped (optional)

1. Preheat the oven to 400°F.

2. Halve the zucchini lengthwise, and use a spoon to scrape out and discard the middle of each half make room for the filling. Place the hollowed zucchini in a 9-by-13-inch baking dish.

3. In large bowl, mix to combine the ricotta and 1 cup of mozzarella with the Parmesan and spinach. Season with salt and pepper.

4. Fill the zucchini with the cheese mixture, and top with the marinara sauce and the remaining 1 cup of mozzarella cheese.

5. Bake for 25 to 30 minutes, until the cheese is melted and the zucchini is tender.

6. Garnish with the basil (if using) and serve.

VARIATION TIP *This is a flexible recipe. Add cooked, crumbled sausage to the cheese filling, or use Alfredo Sauce (page 126) instead of marinara sauce.*

MACRONUTRIENTS **51% FAT**, 31% PROTEIN, 18% CARBS

PER SERVING Calories: 319; Total Fat: 18g; Saturated Fat: 11g; Protein: 24g; Total Carbs: 15g; Fiber: 3g; Net Carbs: 12g; Cholesterol: 58mg

Mac 'n' Cheese

Macaroni and cheese is a well-loved family staple, and now you can make it keto-friendly. You might even like this remake better than the original. It's definitely better for you.

Prep time | 10 minutes   *Cook time* | 20 minutes

NUT-FREE, EGG-FREE, VEGETARIAN

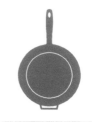

Serves 6

1 cup heavy (whipping) cream

4 ounces cream cheese

2 teaspoons prepared mustard

1½ cups shredded sharp Cheddar cheese, divided

3 cups cauliflower florets, boiled for 5 minutes and drained

1 teaspoon garlic powder

Pinch salt

Pinch freshly ground black pepper

1. Preheat the oven to 375°F.

2. In a large cast iron skillet over medium heat, bring the heavy cream to a simmer. Add the cream cheese and mustard, and whisk until smooth.

3. Stir in 1 cup of shredded Cheddar, and stir until melted. Add the cauliflower, garlic powder, salt, and pepper, and stir until the cheese mixture coats the cauliflower.

4. Sprinkle the remaining 1 cup of cheese over the top, and transfer the skillet to the oven. Bake for 15 to 20 minutes, or until the cheese is browned.

5. Serve hot.

MACRONUTRIENTS **81% FAT,** 12% PROTEIN, 7% CARBS

PER SERVING Calories: 330; Total Fat: 30g; Saturated Fat: 19g; Protein: 10g; Total Carbs: 5g; Fiber: 1g; Net Carbs: 4g; Cholesterol: 105mg

Stuffed Portobello Mushrooms

There's no better way to eat your veggies. This recipe is essentially a rich, delicious spinach-and-artichoke dip baked in mushrooms. How could it not be amazing?

Prep time | 10 minutes   *Cook time* | 25 minutes

NUT-FREE, EGG-FREE, VEGETARIAN

Serves 4

Olive oil cooking spray (optional)

4 large portobello mushrooms, stemmed

1 tablespoon olive oil

Salt

Freshly ground black pepper

1 (10-ounce) package frozen chopped spinach, thawed and drained

1 (14-ounce) can artichoke hearts, drained and chopped

4 ounces cream cheese, at room temperature

¼ cup sour cream

½ cup shredded mozzarella cheese

1 teaspoon garlic powder

¼ cup grated Parmesan cheese

1. Preheat the oven to 450°F. Line a sheet pan with aluminum foil or spray with cooking spray.

2. Rub the mushrooms with the olive oil, and season them with salt and pepper. Place them on the prepared sheet pan and bake for 10 minutes to soften.

3. In a medium bowl, mix to combine the spinach, artichokes, cream cheese, sour cream, mozzarella, and garlic powder, and season with salt and pepper.

4. Divide the mixture among the partially cooked mushrooms, and sprinkle the mushroom caps and filling with the grated Parmesan cheese. Bake for an additional 10 to 15 minutes, until the filling is bubbling.

5. Serve hot.

VARIATION TIP *If you're not a mushroom fan, just make the filling and use it as a dip with celery sticks or zucchini chips.*

MACRONUTRIENTS 65% FAT, 18% PROTEIN, 17% CARBS

PER SERVING Calories: 270; Total Fat: 20g; Saturated Fat: 10g; Protein: 13g; Total Carbs: 12g; Fiber: 6g; Net Carbs: 7g; Cholesterol: 51mg

Zucchini Pesto Noodles

The scent of basil is always enticing. Here it flavors a low-carb take on pesto pasta made with zucchini noodles. Go ahead and get creative with how you spiralize or slice your zucchini. As always, a good-quality sharp knife will make the job quick and easy.

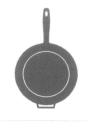

Prep time | 10 minutes *Cook time* | 10 minutes

EGG-FREE, VEGETARIAN, UNDER 30 MINUTES

Serves 4

1 tablespoon olive oil

4 zucchini, cut or spiralized
   into noodles

2 tablespoons pesto

4 ounces cherry tomatoes (about
   5 cherry tomatoes), halved

8 ounces small mozzarella balls, halved

6 basil leaves, chopped

Salt

Freshly ground black pepper

1. In a large skillet over medium heat, heat the olive oil. Add the zucchini noodles. Cook, stirring occasionally, for 3 to 4 minutes, until the zucchini is tender. Drain off any excess liquid.

2. Add the pesto, tomatoes, mozzarella, and basil, season with salt and pepper, and toss to mix. Cook for 2 to 3 minutes longer, until the cheese is melted.

3. Serve immediately.

VARIATION TIP *Spaghetti squash can stand in for the zucchini as another healthy replacement for standard high-carb noodles. You don't even need a spiralizer or any special tool to prepare it. Halve the squash, scoop out the seeds, and bake it cut-side down at 425°F until tender, 30 minutes to an hour depending on the size. Once cooked and halved widthwise, the inside of the squash can be scraped with a fork, and the noodles appear like magic.*

MACRONUTRIENTS **63% FAT,** 22% PROTEIN, 15% CARBS

PER SERVING Calories: 221; Total Fat: 16g; Saturated Fat: 7g; Protein: 12g; Total Carbs: 8g; Fiber: 3g; Net Carbs: 5g; Cholesterol: 41mg

Sautéed Cabbage

Cabbage is often overlooked and gets pushed to the back of the fridge; I know it did in my refrigerator until I went keto. But now I know that cabbage is endlessly versatile. This simple preparation can complement any meal.

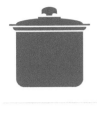

Prep time | 5 minutes   *Cook time* | 15 minutes

DAIRY-FREE, NUT-FREE, EGG-FREE, PALEO, VEGETARIAN, UNDER 30 MINUTES

Serves 4

¼ cup (½ stick) salted butter or ghee
1 head cabbage, chopped
3 tablespoons apple cider vinegar
Salt
Freshly ground black pepper

1. In a large stockpot (I love using my cast iron pot) over medium heat, melt the butter. Add the shredded cabbage and cook, stirring occasionally, until the cabbage is tender. I like my cabbage to still have a little crunch, so I cook it 10 to 12 minutes. If you want yours more tender, cook it a few minutes longer.

2. Add the vinegar, season with salt and pepper, and serve hot.

VARIATION TIP *You can really change the flavor of this simple dish by adding different spices. I like it with cumin, coriander, and/or crushed red pepper. Go ahead and experiment with other flavors that you like.*

MACRONUTRIENTS **63% FAT**, 7% PROTEIN, 30% CARBS

PER SERVING Calories: 158; Total Fat: 12g; Saturated Fat: 17g; Protein: 3g, Total Carbs: 12g; Fiber: 5g; Net Carbs: 7g; Cholesterol: 31mg

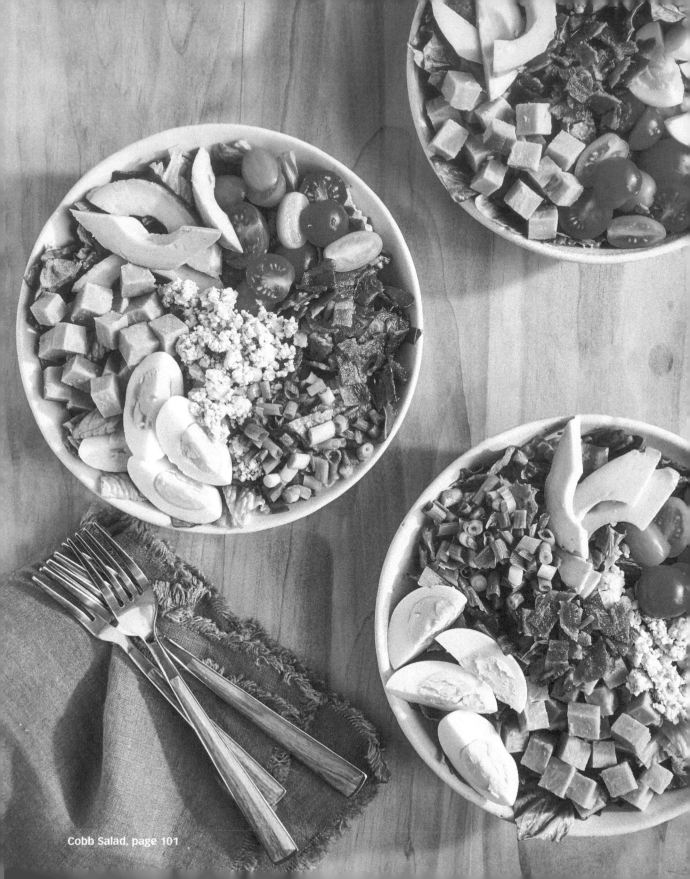

Cobb Salad, page 101

CHAPTER

7

HEARTY
SALADS

Wedge Salad

Salads are ideal for staying on track with your nutritional goals because they are so simple, versatile, and easy to make. This one is especially simple, but it has tons of flavor from the classic combination of bacon and blue cheese.

Prep time | 10 minutes

NUT-FREE, EGG-FREE, UNDER 30 MINUTES

Serves 4

1 head iceberg lettuce, quartered

8 tablespoons blue cheese dressing, divided (I like the Primal Kitchen brand)

3 scallions, white and green parts, chopped

1 cup cherry tomatoes, halved

1 cup crumbled blue cheese

8 pieces Perfectly Cooked Bacon (page 130)

Arrange the lettuce wedges on 4 plates, and drizzle each wedge with 2 tablespoons of blue cheese dressing. Top each with the scallions, tomatoes, cheese, and bacon. Serve immediately.

VARIATION TIP *To make this more of a meal, add chopped hardboiled eggs, grilled chicken, or diced avocado to this salad. I also like to add a splash of balsamic vinegar along with the blue cheese dressing.*

MACRONUTRIENTS **75% FAT,** 17% PROTEIN, 8% CARBS

PER SERVING Calories: 384; Total Fat: 32g; Saturated Fat: 11g; Protein: 15g; Total Carbs: 9g; Fiber: 3g; Net Carbs: 6g; Cholesterol: 52mg

Greek Cucumber Salad

Feta is a Greek cheese made from sheep's and goat's milk. With a distinctive salty, bold taste, feta gives big flavor to simple dishes. I add it to roasted beets, low-carb pizza, and hamburgers and serve it on meat and cheese platters for parties. Here it adds tons of flavor to a simple Greek-style cucumber salad with olives, red onions, and sliced salami or pepperoni.

Serves 6

Prep time | **15 minutes**

NUT-FREE, EGG-FREE, UNDER 30 MINUTES

½ cup olive oil or avocado oil

2 tablespoons red wine vinegar

1 teaspoon dried oregano

1 teaspoon garlic salt

Pinch salt

Pinch freshly ground black pepper

4 cucumbers, peeled and sliced into rounds, then into quarters

4 tomatoes, diced

1 red onion, thinly sliced

2 cups black olives, pitted and sliced

1 cup feta cheese, crumbled

2 cups sliced salami or pepperoni, slices halved

1. In a small bowl, whisk together the olive oil, vinegar, oregano, garlic salt, salt, and pepper.

2. In a large bowl, toss together the cucumbers, tomatoes, onion, olives, cheese, and salami.

3. Pour the dressing over the top, and toss until everything is evenly coated.

4. Serve immediately.

MAKE IT PALEO *Leave out the feta cheese and add diced avocado and freshly squeezed lemon juice instead.*

MACRONUTRIENTS **84% FAT**, 8% PROTEIN, 8% CARBS

PER SERVING Calories: 590; Total Fat: 55g; Saturated Fat: 15g; Protein: 12g; Total Carbs: 12g; Fiber: 2g; Net Carbs: 10g; Cholesterol: 69mg

Chopped Salad with Avocado-Lime Dressing

I didn't realize how many ways you can incorporate avocado into your diet until after I started eating more healthy fats. One of my favorite ways to enjoy avocado is right out of the shell with Himalayan salt and balsamic vinegar. It brings rich creaminess to this homemade avocado-lime dressing, too.

Serves 6

Prep time | **15 minutes**

NUT-FREE, EGG-FREE, UNDER 30 MINUTES

FOR THE DRESSING

1 avocado, plus more if needed
1 cup cilantro leaves, chopped
2 garlic cloves, peeled
½ cup sour cream
3 tablespoons olive oil
1 tablespoon apple cider vinegar
1 tablespoon freshly squeezed
   lime juice
1 teaspoon salt
½ teaspoon garlic powder
½ teaspoon ground cumin
½ teaspoon freshly ground black pepper
1 jalapeño pepper, seeded and
   minced (optional)
Heavy (whipping) cream, for thickening,
   if needed

FOR THE SALAD

1 head romaine lettuce, chopped
8 strips Perfectly Cooked Bacon
   (page 130), crumbled
1 pound cooked and shredded skinless
   chicken breast meat
1 tomato, diced
½ cup crumbled blue cheese or
   feta cheese
1 avocado, cubed

TO MAKE THE DRESSING

In a food processor or blender, combine the avocado, cilantro, garlic, sour cream, olive oil, vinegar, lime juice, salt, garlic powder, cumin, pepper, and jalapeño (if using). Process until smooth. If the dressing is too thick, you can add a bit of water. If it is too thin, add a bit more avocado or a bit of cream.

TO MAKE THE SALAD

Assemble the salads by arranging the chopped lettuce, bacon, chicken, tomatoes, cheese, and avocado on 6 serving plates. Top each with the dressing and serve immediately.

MAKE AHEAD *The avocado-lime dressing will keep for up to a week in an airtight jar in the refrigerator.*

MAKE IT PALEO *To make this dish paleo, substitute a second avocado for the sour cream in the dressing recipe and skip the cheese on the salad.*

MACRONUTRIENTS **67% FAT,** 25% PROTEIN, 8% CARBS

PER SERVING Calories: 374; Total Fat: 28g; Saturated Fat: 9g; Protein: 23g; Total Carbs: 8g; Fiber: 5g; Net Carbs: 3g; Cholesterol: 70mg

Avocado Caprese Salad

The combination of these flavors—avocados, tomatoes, mozzarella, fresh basil, and balsamic vinegar—is one of my very favorites. Whenever I went to my dad's restaurant, he'd put together a caprese salad for me because it was my favorite thing on the menu.

Prep time | 15 minutes

Serves 4

NUT-FREE, EGG-FREE, VEGETARIAN, UNDER 30 MINUTES

2 avocados, cubed

1 cup cherry tomatoes, halved

8 ounces mozzarella balls, halved or quartered

2 tablespoons finely chopped fresh basil

2 tablespoons olive oil

2 tablespoons balsamic vinegar

1 tablespoon salt

Freshly ground black pepper

In a salad bowl, gently toss together the avocados, tomatoes, cheese, basil, olive oil, vinegar, and salt until combined well. Season with pepper and serve immediately.

INGREDIENT TIP *Even though you won't get the full flavor of basil when using dried basil, you can use it in place of fresh if it's your only option. A tablespoon of fresh basil is equivalent to 1 teaspoon of dried.*

MACRONUTRIENTS **74% FAT,** 17% PROTEIN, 9% CARBS

PER SERVING Calories: 358g; Total Fat: 30g; Saturated Fat: 10g; Protein: 14g; Total Carbs: 9g; Fiber: 5g; Net Carbs: 4g; Cholesterol: 44mg

Avocado Salad with Hardboiled Eggs

Eggs and avocados are both superfoods, and they're staples of the low-carb lifestyle. Together they make a perfect meal any time of the day, breakfast, lunch, or dinner. This creamy salad is easy to throw together and provides lots of versatility. You can serve it over greens, in a lettuce wrap, or just on its own.

Serves 2

Prep time | 10 minutes

DAIRY-FREE, NUT-FREE, PALEO, UNDER 30 MINUTES, VEGETARIAN

2 avocados

1 tablespoon freshly squeezed lemon juice

1 teaspoon salt

½ teaspoon freshly ground black pepper

½ teaspoon garlic powder

4 Hardboiled Eggs (page 127), peeled and diced

½ cup chopped celery

¼ cup finely chopped onion or scallions, white and green parts

1. In a medium bowl, mash the avocados with the lemon juice, salt, pepper, and garlic powder, and mix to combine.

2. Gently fold in the eggs, celery, and onion and serve immediately.

VARIATION TIP *You can really play around with this salad. Try adding canned chicken or tuna for a convenient twist. To make this salad creamier, add a tablespoon or two of Mayonnaise (recipe on page 122).*

MACRONUTRIENTS **72% FAT,** 13% PROTEIN, 15% CARBS

PER SERVING Calories: 445; Total Fat: 36g; Saturated Fat: 7g; Protein: 16g; Total Carbs: 17g; Fiber: 13g; Net Carbs: 5g; Cholesterol: 372mg

Cobb Salad

Cobb salads make a great ketogenic meal. They are loaded with healthy fats and flavorful tidbits that make them much more than mere side salads. Having your protein and hardboiled eggs prepped will really cut down on your weeknight meal prep and is the key to quick recipes like this one. Serve this salad with Dairy-Free Ranch Dressing (page 124) or your favorite low-carb bottled dressing.

Serves 4

Prep time | 10 minutes

NUT-FREE, UNDER 30 MINUTES

4 cups chopped romaine lettuce

6 pieces Perfectly Cooked Bacon (page 130), crumbled

4 Hardboiled Eggs (page 127), peeled and sliced

2 cups cubed ham

1 cup crumbled blue cheese

2 avocados, sliced

1 cup cherry tomatoes, sliced

3 scallions, white and green parts, chopped

Dairy-Free Ranch Dressing (page 124) or your favorite low-carb store-bought dressing

Divide the lettuce evenly among 4 large salad bowls. Top each with the bacon, eggs, ham, cheese, avocados, tomatoes, and scallions, arranging the ingredients decoratively on top. Top with dressing and serve immediately.

VARIATION TIP *Don't stress if you don't have any ham in the fridge; you can use leftover chicken, shrimp, or another protein.*

MACRONUTRIENTS **64% FAT**, 27% PROTEIN, 9% CARBS

PER SERVING Calories: 529; Total Fat: 38g; Saturated Fat: 11g; Protein: 36g; Total Carbs: 12g; Fiber: 7g; Net Carbs: 5g; Cholesterol: 262mg

Hot Spinach Salad

Here, bacon grease (aka liquid gold) is a key ingredient in a tasty, warm dressing that wilts the spinach just so when you toss it with the salad. Don't forget to store any leftover bacon grease in the fridge. Use it to fry meats, grease pans, scramble eggs, caramelize onions, or roast vegetables.

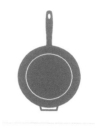

Serves 6

Prep time | 15 minutes   *Cook time* | 10 minutes

NUT-FREE, UNDER 30 MINUTES

---

12 uncured bacon slices

3 tablespoons apple cider vinegar

1 tablespoon sugar substitute (such as Swerve)

1 teaspoon Dijon mustard

6 cups fresh spinach

6 Hardboiled Eggs (page 127), peeled and sliced

2 cups sliced mushrooms

1 red onion, thinly sliced

1½ cups shredded Swiss cheese

1. In a large skillet over medium-low heat, cook the bacon to your desired crispiness, or for about 8 minutes. Transfer to a paper towel–lined plate, and crumble when cool.

2. Return the skillet with the bacon drippings to the burner. Over low heat, continuously whisk the vinegar, sweetener, and mustard until the sweetener is dissolved and the dressing is warm, about 2 minutes.

3. To assemble the salads, divide the spinach, bacon crumbles, eggs, mushrooms, onion, and cheese evenly among 4 salad bowls.

4. When ready to serve, spoon the warm bacon dressing over the top and serve immediately.

VARIATION TIP *A handful of fresh sliced strawberries, tossed on after the dressing has been added, goes surprisingly well with the flavors in this salad. Sautéing the mushrooms and onion in the bacon grease before making the dressing will take this salad to the next level.*

MACRONUTRIENTS **62% FAT**, 30% PROTEIN, 8% CARBS

PER SERVING Calories: 265; Total Fat: 18g; Saturated Fat: 9g; Protein: 19g; Total Carbs: 5g; Fiber: 1g; Net Carbs: 4g; Cholesterol: 221mg

Chicken Caesar Salad

This classic salad has become a staple at my house and pairs well with just about anything. You can keep a Caesar salad very basic or dress it up by adding avocado, Hardboiled Eggs (page 127), anchovies, grilled chicken, shrimp, Perfectly Cooked Bacon (page 130), grilled steak, and/or tomatoes and serve it as a formal dinner salad.

Serves 4

Prep time | 10 minutes

NUT-FREE, EGG-FREE, UNDER 30 MINUTES

1 head romaine lettuce, chopped

4 (4-ounce) boneless, skinless chicken breasts, cooked and cubed

½ cup Caesar Dressing (page 123)

½ cup grated Parmesan cheese, divided

1. In a large salad bowl, toss together the lettuce, chicken, dressing, and ¼ cup of Parmesan cheese.

2. Add any desired toppings, plate, and serve with the remaining ¼ cup of Parmesan cheese sprinkled on top.

INGREDIENT TIP *Homemade dressing made from scratch is the ideal choice, but that's not always feasible. When grabbing a bottled dressing from the store, be sure to read the label carefully. Keep an eye out for sugar and carbs, which can be very, very sneaky.*

MACRONUTRIENTS **53% FAT**, 39% PROTEIN, 8% CARBS

PER SERVING Calories: 343; Total Fat: 20g; Saturated Fat: 5g; Protein: 33g; Total Carbs: 7g; Fiber: 3g; Net Carbs: 4g; Cholesterol: 75mg

Taco Salad

When I order taco salads out and ask for no tortilla, no beans, and no rice, I get some confused looks. But I really don't miss those things living low carb, especially with simple salads like this one. The seasoned meat, cheese, avocado, and sour cream are the best parts anyway.

Prep time | 15 minutes

Serves 6

NUT-FREE, UNDER 30 MINUTES

FOR THE SALAD

6 cups chopped romaine lettuce

1 pound cooked ground beef

1 tomato, diced

1 cup shredded sharp Cheddar cheese

FOR TOPPING

1 avocado, sliced

½ cup low-carb salsa

½ cup sour cream

Freshly squeezed lime juice

Salt

Freshly ground black pepper

Chopped cilantro leaves, for serving

1 cup Dairy-Free Ranch Dressing
  (page 124)

1. In a large salad bowl, toss together the lettuce, prepared meat, tomato, and cheese until combined.

2. Divide the salad among individual bowls, arrange the toppings in dishes on the counter or table, and let each diner top their salad with the desired remaining ingredients.

VARIATION TIP *Try switching up the protein with shredded cooked chicken or pork.*

MACRONUTRIENTS **69% FAT**, 20% PROTEIN, 11% CARBS

PER SERVING Calories: 467; Total Fat: 36g; Saturated Fat: 11g; Protein: 23g; Total Carbs: 12g; Fiber: 4g; Net Carbs: 8g; Cholesterol: 85mg

Flank Steak Salad

When in doubt, go for a salad! If it's one that's topped with flank steak, avocado, and feta cheese, you'll be glad you did. Salads are a great way to stay keto when dining out and are quick and easy to put together at home.

Prep time | 10 minutes   *Cook time* | 10 minutes

NUT-FREE, EGG-FREE, UNDER 30 MINUTES

Serves 4

¼ cup plus 2 tablespoons olive oil, divided

12 ounces flank steak

Salt

Freshly ground black pepper

6 cups fresh spinach

2 avocados, cubed

4 ounces feta cheese, crumbled

Juice of 1 lemon

1. Set the broiler to high.

2. Rub 2 tablespoons of olive oil all over the steak, and season on both sides with salt and pepper.

3. Place the steak on a broiler pan or sheet pan and cook under the broiler to your desired doneness (3 to 4 minutes per side for medium-rare).

4. Transfer the steak to a cutting board, and let it rest for 5 to 10 minutes.

5. While the steak is resting, in a salad bowl, toss together the spinach, avocado, and feta cheese. Add the remaining ¼ cup of olive oil and the lemon juice, season with salt and pepper, and toss to mix well. Divide the salad evenly among 4 serving bowls.

6. Slice the steak across the grain into thin strips, top each salad with one-quarter of the meat, and serve.

VARIATION TIP *Try this recipe with homemade or store-bought low-carb blue cheese or Caesar dressing.*

MACRONUTRIENTS **76% FAT,** 17% PROTEIN, 7% CARBS

PER SERVING Calories: 541; Total Fat: 46g; Saturated Fat: 12g; Protein: 24g; Total Carbs: 10g; Fiber: 7g; Net Carbs: 3g; Cholesterol: 68mg

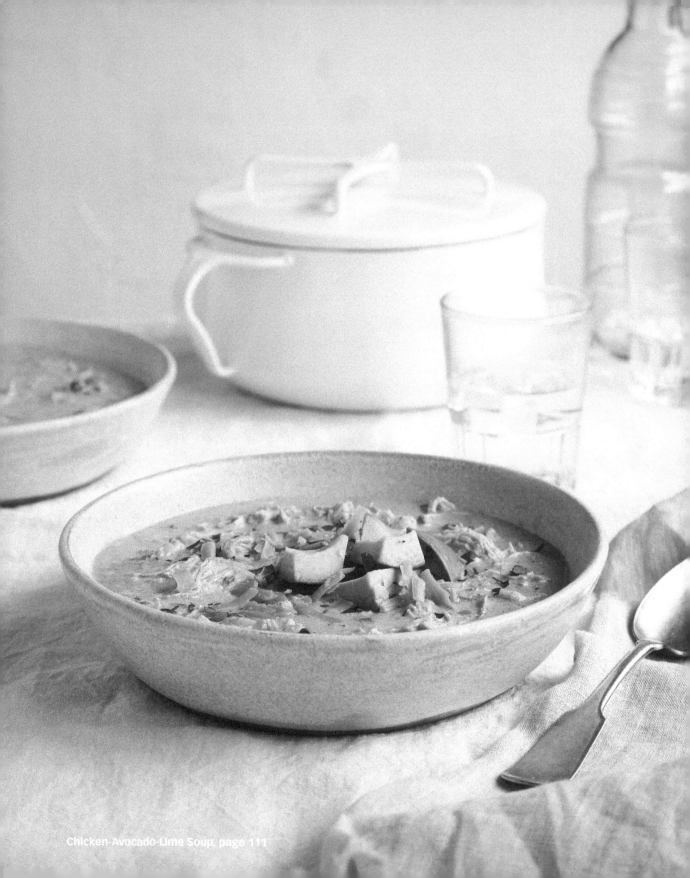

Chicken-Avocado-Lime Soup, page 111

CHAPTER

8

SOUPS
& STEWS

Tomato-Basil Soup

Nothing says comfort like an old-fashioned tomato-basil soup. If you don't have an immersion blender, pour the soup (carefully) into a countertop blender and blend until smooth. Make sure to remove the center fill cap from the blender lid and cover it with a hand towel so the steam can escape while you blend. Serve the soup topped with additional chopped basil and freshly grated Parmesan cheese, if you like.

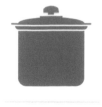

Serves 6

Prep time | 10 minutes   *Cook time* | 25 minutes

NUT-FREE, EGG-FREE, VEGETARIAN

---

2 tablespoons olive oil

1 yellow onion, diced

2 garlic cloves, minced

2 (28-ounce) cans whole peeled tomatoes in their juice

2 cups vegetable broth

½ cup salted butter

½ cup chopped basil leaves, divided

1 cup heavy (whipping) cream

Salt

Freshly ground black pepper

1. In a large stockpot over medium heat, heat the olive oil. Add the onion and garlic and cook, stirring frequently, until browned, about 5 minutes.

2. Add the tomatoes with their juice, broth, and butter and bring to a boil. Reduce the heat to low and simmer, uncovered, for 20 minutes. Add the basil and purée the soup in the stockpot with an immersion blender.

3. Stir in the cream, season with salt and pepper, and serve hot.

MAKE IT PALEO *To make this dish Paleo, use coconut cream in place of the heavy cream and ghee in place of the butter.*

MACRONUTRIENTS **84% FAT,** 4% PROTEIN, 12% CARBS

PER SERVING (without Parmesan) Calories: 371; Total Fat: 36g; Saturated Fat: 20g; Protein: 4g; Total Carbs: 11g; Fiber: 2g; Net Carbs: 9g; Cholesterol: 97mg

Broccoli-Cheese Soup

This delicious soup is a classic. It's loaded with healthy broccoli and two kinds of cheese to give it lots of flavor and heft. Serve this on a chilly winter evening or put it in a thermos for a portable lunch that will keep you warm on a cold day.

Prep time | 10 minutes   *Cook time* | 20 minutes

NUT-FREE, EGG-FREE

Serves 6

2 tablespoons salted butter

1 yellow onion, diced

1 cup diced celery

4 cups broccoli florets

3 cups chicken broth

1 cup heavy (whipping) cream

2 cups shredded Cheddar cheese, plus more for serving

1 cup shredded Swiss cheese, plus more for serving

1 teaspoon garlic powder

Pinch salt

Pinch freshly ground black pepper

1. In a large stockpot over medium heat, melt the butter. Add the onion and celery and cook, stirring frequently, until browned and softened, 4 to 5 minutes.

2. Add the broccoli, broth, and cream to the pot and bring to a simmer, stirring constantly (you don't want the cream to burn). Reduce the heat to low and simmer for 10 minutes, or until the broccoli is cooked through. Stir in the cheeses and garlic powder until well combined and the cheese is melted, about 5 minutes.

3. Season with salt and pepper and serve immediately with extra shredded cheese on top.

INGREDIENT TIP *If this soup isn't thick enough for your taste, add a little xanthan gum as a thickener. A little bit of this powder goes a long way. You can buy it at health food stores or online.*

MACRONUTRIENTS 75% FAT, 17% PROTEIN, 8% CARBS

PER SERVING Calories: 385; Total Fat: 32g; Saturated Fat: 20g; Protein: 17g; Total Carbs: 8g; Fiber: 3g; Net Carbs: 5g; Cholesterol: 110mg

Clam Chowder

I always imagined clam chowder to be very labor intensive, and that's totally not the case. With the right ingredients on hand, it doesn't take much thought or time at all to get a creamy bowl of clam chowder on the dinner table.

Prep time | 10 minutes   *Cook time* | 30 minutes

NUT-FREE, EGG-FREE

Serves 8

1 tablespoon olive oil

8 uncured bacon slices, cut into 1-inch pieces

1 yellow onion, diced

2 cups diced celery

4 garlic cloves, minced

2 cups chicken broth

1 head cauliflower, chopped into florets

1 (8-ounce) bottle clam juice

1 teaspoon salt

½ teaspoon chopped fresh thyme

½ teaspoon freshly ground black pepper

2 cups heavy (whipping) cream

½ teaspoon xanthan gum

3 (10-ounce) cans clams, drained, and chopped if needed

1. In a large stockpot over medium heat, heat the olive oil. Add the bacon and cook it to your desired crispiness, about 8 minutes. Transfer the bacon to a paper towel–lined plate. Add the onion, celery, and garlic to the remaining bacon grease, and cook until tender, about 5 minutes.

2. Add the broth, cauliflower, clam juice, salt, thyme, and pepper, and bring to boil. Reduce the heat and simmer for about 15 minutes, or until the cauliflower is tender.

3. Add the cream and xanthan gum to the soup and bring to a boil. Cook, stirring constantly, for 1 to 2 minutes, or until the soup thickens.

4. Fold in the clams and bacon just before serving. Serve hot.

INGREDIENT TIP *Xanthan gum is a specialty item that can be found in health food stores or at online retailers. It's a fine powder that acts as a thickener in soups, sauces, and shakes. A little xanthan gum goes a long way. Add it ¼ teaspoon at a time until the soup reaches desired consistency.*

MACRONUTRIENTS **63% FAT**, 22% PROTEIN, 15% CARBS

PER SERVING Calories: 388; Total Fat: 27g; Saturated Fat: 15g; Protein: 21g; Total Carbs: 15g; Fiber: 3g; Net Carbs: 12g; Cholesterol: 128mg

Chicken-Avocado-Lime Soup

Reheating this soup after a few days is what convinced me to love leftovers. Like with many soups, the distinct flavors meld and get better with time. Hold off on adding in the avocado until you are ready to serve the soup.

Prep time | 15 minutes   *Cook time* | 30 minutes

NUT-FREE, EGG-FREE

Serves 8

3 tablespoons olive oil or avocado oil

2 jalapeño peppers, seeded and minced

4 garlic cloves, minced

1 yellow onion, diced

1 teaspoon ground cumin

1 teaspoon chili powder

1 teaspoon garlic salt

Salt

Freshly ground black pepper

4 cups chicken broth

3 tomatoes, diced, or 1 (14.5-ounce) can diced tomatoes

1½ pounds boneless, skinless chicken breasts

8 ounces cream cheese, cubed

2 cups cilantro leaves, chopped

Juice of 2 limes

1 cup shredded sharp Cheddar cheese

2 avocados, cubed

1. In a large stockpot over medium heat, heat the olive oil. Add the jalapeños, garlic, and onion and cook, stirring frequently, until the onion is soft and translucent, 4 to 6 minutes.

2. Stir in the cumin, chili powder, and garlic salt, and season with salt and pepper. Add the broth and tomatoes, and bring to a boil. Add the chicken breasts, and reduce the heat to low. Cover and simmer for 15 to 20 minutes, or until the chicken is cooked through. Transfer the chicken to a cutting board, shred the meat using two forks, and return it to the pot.

3. Add the cream cheese, cilantro, and lime juice and simmer, stirring, until the cream cheese is melted and combined, about 5 minutes.

4. Serve topped with shredded cheese and avocado.

MACRONUTRIENTS **65% FAT**, 25% PROTEIN, 10% CARBS

PER SERVING Calories: 402; Total Fat: 39g; Saturated Fat: 12g; Protein: 26g; Total Carbs: 11g; Fiber: 4g; Net Carbs: 7g; Cholesterol: 95mg

Chicken and Zucchini Noodle Soup

Your family will never know this delicious soup only took around 30 minutes to make from start to finish. This is a great recipe to use up leftover chicken—you can even use the bones to make the broth. Having the zucchini noodles pre-prepped will cut down on the preparation time even more, and you'll have "chicken-zoodle" soup in no time.

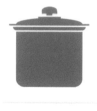

Serves 8

Prep time | 10 minutes   *Cook time* | 25 minutes

DAIRY-FREE, NUT-FREE, EGG-FREE, PALEO

---

4 tablespoons olive oil, divided

2 pounds skin-on, bone-in chicken thighs

Salt

Freshly ground black pepper

1 yellow onion, chopped

2 garlic cloves, minced

2 cups chopped celery

4 cups chicken broth

2 bay leaves

1 teaspoon chopped fresh thyme

4 zucchini, cut or spiralized into noodles

1. In a large stockpot over medium heat, heat 2 tablespoons of olive oil. Pat the chicken thighs dry with paper towels, and season with salt and pepper. Add the chicken to the pot, skin-side down, and cook for 3 to 5 minutes on each side, until nicely browned. Transfer the partially cooked thighs to a plate and set aside.

2. In the same pot, heat the remaining 2 tablespoons of olive oil and add the onion, garlic, and celery. Season with salt and pepper. Cook for 3 to 4 minutes, or until browned.

3. Add the chicken, broth, bay leaves, thyme, and zucchini, and bring to a boil. Reduce the heat to low, and simmer for 10 minutes.

4. Transfer the chicken to another plate, and pull the meat from the bones. Shred the meat, and return it to the pot.

5. Remove the bay leaves and serve hot.

INGREDIENT TIP *Bay leaves release their flavor during slow cooking, so the longer the better. Using bay leaves in soups, casseroles, and stews is a great way to add flavor. Always remember to leave the leaf whole and remove before eating.*

MACRONUTRIENTS **54% FAT**, 36% PROTEIN, 10% CARBS

PER SERVING Calories: 285; Total Fat: 17g; Saturated Fat: 4g; Protein: 26g; Total Carbs: 7g; Fiber: 2g; Net Carbs: 5g; Cholesterol: 92mg

Cauliflower-Ham Chowder

Cauliflower is a good replacement for potatoes. Once it's cooked and mashed or puréed, it has the same ability to thicken up soups and sauces. This is a great soup when it's cold outside and you want something warm, filling, and comforting. And because it is made in the slow cooker, you can get it ready to go in the morning before you leave for work. When you come home, all you have to do is pop in the cauliflower and relax for 30 minutes until it is ready.

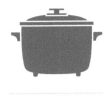

Serves 8

Prep time | 10 minutes   *Cook time* | 8 hours 30 minutes

NUT-FREE, EGG-FREE, UNDER 30 MINUTES

3 cups diced ham

½ cup heavy (whipping) cream

3 cups chicken broth

2 cups shredded sharp white Cheddar cheese

1 teaspoon garlic salt

1 teaspoon onion powder

1 bay leaf

Salt

Freshly ground black pepper

6 cups cauliflower florets

1. In the slow cooker, combine the ham, cream, broth, cheese, garlic salt, onion powder, and bay leaf. Season with salt and pepper. Cover and cook on low for 6 to 8 hours.

2. Add the cauliflower and cook for and additional 30 minutes on high, or until the cauliflower is tender.

3. Remove the bay leaf and serve hot.

VARIATION TIP *If you prefer a creamier soup, use an immersion blender or countertop blender (carefully) to blend the soup to your desired consistency.*

MACRONUTRIENTS **59% FAT**, 31% PROTEIN, 10% CARBS

PER SERVING Calories: 310; Total Fat: 21g; Saturated Fat: 11g; Protein: 23g; Total Carbs: 8g; Fiber: 2g; Net Carbs: 6g; Cholesterol: 84mg

Italian Sausage Soup

This soup resembles one you'd eat at a beautiful Italian restaurant rather than in the comfort of your own home. Try adding fresh parsley and grated Parmesan cheese to complete this Italian-inspired soup, or leave out the cheese and use coconut milk instead of heavy cream to make this recipe dairy-free and Paleo.

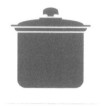

Serves 8

Prep time | 10 minutes   *Cook time* | 25 minutes

NUT-FREE, EGG-FREE

1 pound bulk sweet or hot
  Italian sausage

1 yellow onion, chopped

3 garlic cloves, minced

4 cups beef broth

4 cups finely chopped cabbage

1 cup chopped celery

1 teaspoon dried oregano

1 bay leaf

Salt

Freshly ground black pepper

1 cup heavy (whipping) cream or
  full-fat coconut milk

1 teaspoon crushed red pepper flakes

1. In a large stockpot over medium heat, cook the sausage for 2 minutes. Add the onion and garlic, and cook with the sausage until the onion is translucent and the sausage is browned, 3 to 5 minutes more.

2. Add the broth, cabbage, celery, oregano, and bay leaf, season with salt and pepper, and reduce the heat to low. Simmer for 15 minutes. Add the cream and simmer until just heated through.

3. Remove and discard the bay leaf, and serve the soup topped with the crushed red pepper flakes.

MAKE AHEAD *Fill mason jars three-quarters full of prepared soup and freeze with the lids off (to prevent the jars from breaking when the soup expands as it freezes). Put the lids on and store in the freezer for up to 3 months.*

MACRONUTRIENTS **77% FAT,** 15% PROTEIN, 8% CARBS

PER SERVING Calories: 334; Total Fat: 29g; Saturated Fat: 13g; Protein: 12g; Total Carbs: 7g; Fiber: 2g; Net Carbs: 5g; Cholesterol: 83mg

Enchilada Soup

You don't have to miss out on Mexican flavors just because you're doing a keto lifestyle. Just skip the tortillas and refried beans and you're good. Cumin is a common Mexican seasoning and is used in taco seasoning mixes. This soup uses a hefty dose for authentic Mexican flavor.

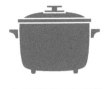

Serves 8

Prep time | 20 minutes   *Cook time* | 6 hours

NUT-FREE, EGG-FREE

FOR THE SOUP

4 boneless, skinless chicken breasts

1 (16-ounce) jar low-carb mild salsa

4 scallions, white and green
    parts, sliced

4 cups chicken broth

1 (4-ounce) can diced green chiles

2 cups shredded pepper Jack cheese

8 ounces cream cheese

1 tablespoon ground cumin

1 tablespoon chili powder

FOR TOPPING

Sliced black olives

Shredded lettuce

Sliced avocado

Shredded cheese

Sour cream

Lime wedges

1. In the slow cooker, combine the chicken, salsa, scallions, broth, chiles, pepper Jack, cream cheese, cumin, and chili powder. Cover and cook on low for 6 to 8 hours.

2. Transfer the chicken breasts to a platter and use two forks to shred the meat. Return the shredded chicken to the pot and serve the soup hot with desired toppings.

VARIATION TIP *This soup works well with seasoned ground beef from the Taco Bar recipe (page 57) instead of chicken breasts. You will need to precook the taco meat before adding it to the slow cooker.*

MACRONUTRIENTS **62% FAT,** 30% PROTEIN, 8% CARBS

PER SERVING Calories: 303; Total Fat: 21g; Saturated Fat: 13g; Protein: 22g; Total Carbs: 6g; Fiber: 1g; Net Carbs: 5g; Cholesterol: 91mg

Slow Cooker Pizza Soup

You can switch this recipe up depending on what type of pizza you love. My favorite kind of pizza is supreme, so this recipe includes sausage, green pepper, olives, mushrooms, pepperoni, and mozzarella cheese. Get creative; you can't mess this up!

Prep time | 15 minutes   *Cook time* | 6 hours

NUT-FREE, EGG-FREE

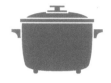

Serves 8

1 pound bulk sweet or hot Italian
  sausage, browned

2 (15-ounce) cans diced
  tomatoes, drained

1 (6-ounce) can tomato paste

2 cups beef broth

2 (8-ounce) packages cream cheese

1 green bell pepper, seeded and diced

6 ounces mushrooms, sliced

1 cup black olives, sliced

1 cup sliced pepperoni

2 tablespoons Italian seasoning

Salt

Freshly ground black pepper

1 cup shredded mozzarella

1. In a slow cooker, combine the sausage, tomatoes, tomato paste, broth, cream cheese, bell pepper, mushrooms, olives, pepperoni, and Italian seasoning, and season with salt and pepper. Stir to combine, cover, and cook on low for 6 to 7 hours.

2. Serve topped with the mozzarella cheese.

MACRONUTRIENTS **74% FAT**, 16% PROTEIN, 10% CARBS

PER SERVING Calories: 507; Total Fat: 42g; Saturated Fat: 22g; Protein: 21g; Total Carbs: 13g; Fiber: 2g; Net Carbs: 11g; Cholesterol: 128mg

Low-Carb Chili

A big pot of spicy, meaty chili is great for serving a crowd, or for serving the family several meals. Like many soups, chili only gets better in the day or two after it is made, so don't be afraid to make a lot and enjoy the leftovers. It may surprise you, but I'm certain you won't miss the beans in this hearty chili. Be sure to have shredded cheese, sour cream, hot sauce, and any other chili toppings you like so that everyone can customize their own bowl.

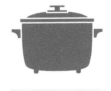

Serves 10

Prep time | 25 minutes   *Cook time* | 4 to 10 hours

DAIRY-FREE, NUT-FREE, EGG-FREE, PALEO

1 pound ground beef, browned

1 pound bulk sausage, browned

1 pound Perfectly Cooked Bacon (page 130), diced

2 cups beef broth

1 cup chopped celery

2 (15-ounce) cans diced tomatoes with juice

1 (6-ounce) can tomato paste

1 (4-ounce) can diced green chiles

2 tablespoons Worcestershire sauce

2 tablespoons chili powder

2 tablespoons ground cumin

2 teaspoon garlic salt

1 teaspoon freshly ground black pepper

1. In the slow cooker, combine the browned beef and sausage with the bacon, broth, celery, tomatoes with their juice, tomato paste, chiles, Worcestershire sauce, chili powder, cumin, garlic salt, and pepper, and stir to combine. Cover and cook on low for 8 to 10 hours or on high for 4 to 6 hours.

2. Serve hot, topped with your favorite toppings.

MAKE AHEAD *This chili freezes and reheats very well, so double the batch when you can.*

MACRONUTRIENTS 58% FAT, 30% PROTEIN, 12% CARBS

PER SERVING Calories: 325; Total Fat: 21g; Saturated Fat: 10g; Protein: 24g; Total Carbs: 10g; Fiber: 2g; Net Carbs: 8g; Cholesterol: 79mg

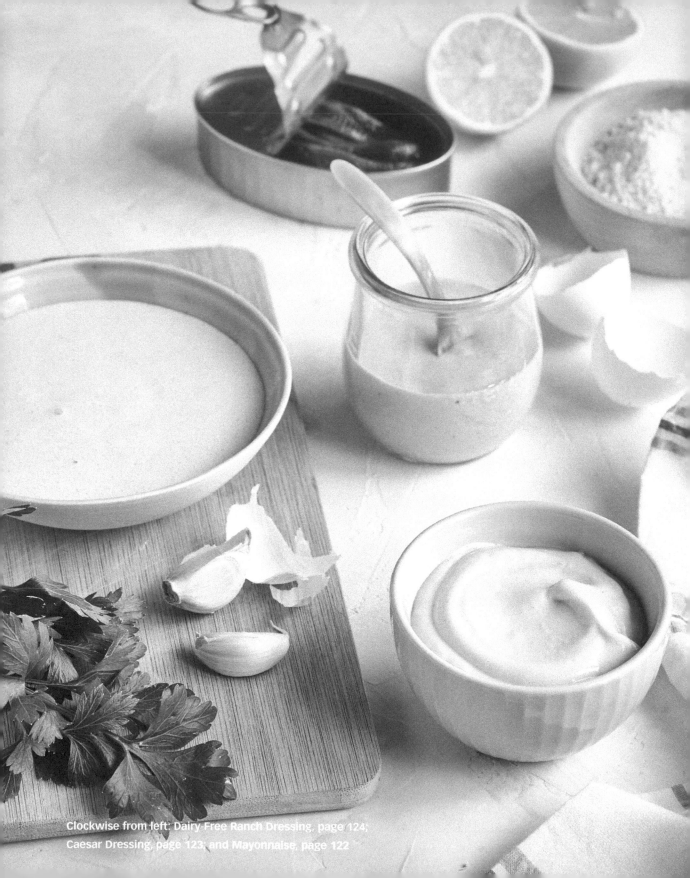

Clockwise from left: Dairy-Free Ranch Dressing, page 124; Caesar Dressing, page 123; and Mayonnaise, page 122

CHAPTER
9

KETO
BASICS

Fat Coffee

Fat coffee is a staple in my ketogenic lifestyle. If I don't start my mornings with a frothy cup of it, my whole day is off, including my macros. You can dress this recipe up or down, and it will keep you satisfied and full of energy for hours. To dress your coffee up, add collagen peptides, ground cinnamon, cocoa powder, sweeteners and/or sugar-free syrups.

Serves 1

Prep time | **5 minutes**

NUT-FREE, EGG-FREE, VEGETARIAN, UNDER 30 MINUTES

1 cup freshly brewed coffee

1 tablespoon salted butter, at room temperature

1 tablespoon coconut oil, melted

1 tablespoon heavy (whipping) cream or full-fat coconut milk

Pour the hot coffee into your blender. Add the butter, oil, and cream and blend for 30 to 60 seconds, until frothy. Serve hot and embrace the fat.

VARIATION TIP *If you aren't a coffee drinker, you can replace coffee with hot tea or brewed cacao nibs. (You can find the nibs online and in most health food stores. I like the Crio Bru brand.)*

MACRONUTRIENTS **98% FAT**, 1% PROTEIN, 1% CARBS

PER SERVING Calories: 271; Total Fat: 31g; Saturated Fat: 22g; Protein: 1g; Total Carbs: 0g; Fiber: 0g; Net Carbs: 0g; Cholesterol: 51mg

Bone Broth

Bone broth should become a staple when you begin your keto-genic journey. It will help your body cope with the adjustment to a keto diet and is very nutrient dense. Bone broth is a great way to replenish the electrolytes you lose by reducing carbs in your diet. When you're feeling low energy or a headache is coming on, sip on warm bone broth for relief.

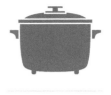

Serves 4

Prep time | 15 minutes   *Cook time* | 8 to 24 hours

DAIRY-FREE, NUT-FREE, EGG-FREE, PALEO

---

3 pounds mixed bones (beef, chicken, or pork)

2 carrots, chopped

4 celery stalks, chopped

2 onions, chopped

2 tablespoons olive oil

2 tablespoons apple cider vinegar

2 whole garlic cloves

1 teaspoon salt

1. In a slow cooker, combine the bones, carrots, celery, onions, olive oil, vinegar, garlic, and salt, and cover completely with water.

2. Cover the slow cooker, and turn it on high. Once the liquid begins to simmer, change the slow cooker setting to low and cook for 8 to 24 hours.

3. Strain the broth through a mesh strainer, and discard the solids.

4. Serve warm or store in mason jars in the refrigerator for up to 4 days or in resealable plastic bags in the freezer for up to a month.

VARIATION TIP *Try adding any fresh herbs or ginger, black peppercorns, and/or bay leaf to the recipe above. There is no wrong way to do bone broth; get creative!*

MACRONUTRIENTS **37% FAT**, 41% PROTEIN, 22% CARBS

PER SERVING (1 cup) Calories 56; Total Fat: 2g; Saturated Fat: 0g; Protein: 5g; Total Carbs: 1g; Fiber: 0g; Net Carbs: 1g; Cholesterol: 0mg

Mayonnaise

This recipe for mayonnaise is simple to make, it can be stored for up to a week, and it makes for a guilt-free addition to just about any dish. Incorporating mayonnaise into your meal is a great way to stay within your fat goals for the day.

Prep time | 10 minutes

DAIRY-FREE, NUT FREE, PALEO, VEGETARIAN, UNDER 30 MINUTES

Makes about 2 cups

2 large egg yolks, at room temperature

2 tablespoons freshly squeezed lemon juice

1 tablespoon apple cider vinegar

1 teaspoon salt

1 teaspoon Dijon mustard

1½ cups olive oil or avocado oil

1. In a food processor, combine the yolks, lemon juice, vinegar, salt, and mustard, and blend for about 30 seconds, or until the mixture thickens.

2. With the food processor on high speed, slowly drizzle in the olive oil in a thin stream until the mixture thickens.

3. Store in a glass jar or airtight container in the refrigerator for up to a week.

ALLERGEN TIP *To make this recipe egg free, replace the egg yolks with 2 tablespoons of coconut oil.*

MACRONUTRIENTS **99% FAT**, 1% PROTEIN, 0% CARBS

PER SERVING Calories: 94; Total Fat: 10g; Saturated Fat: 2g; Protein: 0g; Total Carbs: 0g; Fiber: 0g; Net Carbs: 0g; Cholesterol: 12mg

Caesar Dressing

A few years ago, at a fine Italian restaurant, I ordered a beautiful Caesar salad topped with aged Parmesan cheese and whole anchovies. Until that fancy salad, I was unaware anchovies played such an important role in Caesar salads. My point being, don't let the anchovy paste in the ingredient list scare you away from this recipe. If you have enjoyed a Caesar salad in the past, you've most likely enjoyed anchovies as well. Play around with the amounts and find a balance that satisfies your palate.

Makes 1 cup

Prep time | 10 minutes

NUT-FREE, UNDER 30 MINUTES

2 garlic cloves, smashed

1 teaspoon anchovy paste

2 **egg** yolks

Juice of 1 lemon

1 teaspoon prepared mustard

1 teaspoon Worcestershire sauce

½ cup olive oil or avocado oil

¼ cup grated Parmesan cheese

Salt

Freshly ground black pepper

1. In a large blender, combine the garlic, anchovy paste, egg yolks, lemon juice, mustard, and Worcestershire sauce. Blend for 30 seconds or until the mixture becomes smooth.

2. With the blender running on medium speed, slowly drizzle the olive oil in until the dressing becomes thick and creamy.

3. Stir in the Parmesan cheese, and season generously with salt and pepper.

4. Chill for 30 minutes and serve cold. Store refrigerated in an airtight container for up to a week.

INGREDIENT TIP *Shop for anchovies and anchovy paste near the canned tuna in your grocery store.*

MACRONUTRIENTS **96% FAT,** 4% PROTEIN, 0% CARBS

PER SERVING (1 tablespoon) Calories: 75; Total Fat: 8g; Saturated Fat: 1g; Protein: 1g; Total Carbs: 0g; Fiber: 0g; Net Carbs: 0g; Cholesterol: 24mg

Dairy-Free Ranch Dressing

This ranch dressing is versatile and easy to make. It's delicious added to any salad, spooned over steamed or roasted vegetables, or even used as a marinade for meat or fish. If you are short on time or in a pickle, look for the commercial ranch dressing with the lowest carbs in the refrigerated produce section of your supermarket. I love the vegan ranch by Follow Your Heart. It's high in fat, dairy-free, and super low in carbs.

Makes 1½ cups

Prep time | 10 minutes, plus at least 1 hour to chill

DAIRY-FREE, NUT-FREE, VEGETARIAN

1 cup Mayonnaise (page 122)

½ cup full-fat coconut milk

2 garlic cloves, finely minced

1 tablespoon freshly squeezed lemon juice

1 tablespoon apple cider vinegar

2 tablespoons minced flat-leaf parsley

Salt

Freshly ground black pepper

1. In a blender, combine the mayo, coconut milk, garlic, lemon juice, vinegar, and parsley, and season with salt and pepper. Blend on high for 1 to 2 minutes, until smooth.

2. Chill for at least 1 hour before serving. Store in an airtight container in the refrigerator for up to a week.

ALLERGEN TIP *For an egg-free version, use the egg-free variation of Mayonnaise (page 122).*

MACRONUTRIENTS **96% FAT,** 2% PROTEIN, 3% CARBS

PER SERVING (¼ cup) Calories: 279; Total Fat: 30g; Saturated Fat: 7g; Protein: 1g; Total Carbs: 2g; Fiber: 0g; Net Carbs: 2g; Cholesterol: 10mg

Hollandaise Sauce

You don't need a traditional double boiler for this recipe; using a blender makes it quick and easy to whip up. Hollandaise sauce is perfect over asparagus, poached eggs, and even steaks. It is best to make this sauce right before the meal rather than prep in advance.

Prep time | 10 minutes

NUT-FREE, VEGETARIAN, UNDER 30 MINUTES

Makes about 1½ cups
(Twelve 2-tablespoon servings)

6 large egg yolks
1 tablespoon freshly squeezed
   lemon juice
1 teaspoon salt
Pinch ground cayenne pepper
1 cup (2 sticks) salted butter, melted

1. In a blender, combine the egg yolks, lemon juice, salt, and cayenne. Pulse a few times to mix, and scrape down the sides of the blender with a spatula.

2. With the blender running at medium speed, slowly drizzle the melted butter into the egg mixture. You should notice it has thickened by the time you have added all the butter. Blend for an additional 30 seconds to thicken.

3. Serve immediately.

MAKE IT PALEO *To make this sauce dairy-free instead of vegetarian, use duck fat or lard instead of butter.*

MACRONUTRIENTS **94% FAT**, 6% PROTEIN, 0% CARBS

PER SERVING Calories: 163; Total Fat: 17g; Saturated Fat: 10g; Protein: 2g; Total Carbs: 0g; Fiber: 0g; Net Carbs: 0g; Cholesterol: 133mg

Alfredo Sauce

This rich and creamy sauce is great to have on hand throughout your busy week. I recommend prepping Alfredo sauce and storing it in a mason jar for 4 to 5 days in the refrigerator. I often warm the sauce up in the microwave or on the stovetop and then spoon it over chicken, zucchini noodles, or low-carb shirataki noodles.

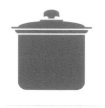

Makes about 3 cups

Prep time | 5 minutes   *Cook time* | 10 minutes

NUT-FREE, EGG-FREE, VEGETARIAN, UNDER 30 MINUTES

½ cup (1 stick) salted butter
2 garlic cloves, minced
1½ cups heavy (whipping) cream
6 ounces cream cheese
1 cup grated Parmesan cheese
Salt
Freshly ground black pepper

1. In a medium saucepan over medium heat, melt the butter and add the garlic. Sauté for 1 to 2 minutes, and then add the cream and the cream cheese.

2. Bring to a simmer and continue to cook, stirring constantly, for 5 to 6 minutes, or until the sauce thickens.

3. Reduce to low heat and add the Parmesan. Season with salt and pepper.

4. Serve hot or let cool to room temperature before storing.

VARIATION TIP *If you prefer a thicker sauce, try stirring ¼ teaspoon of xanthan gum in at the end.*

MACRONUTRIENTS **89% FAT,** 8% PROTEIN, 3% CARBS

PER SERVING (⅓ cup) Calories: 339; Total Fat: 34g; Saturated Fat: 21g; Protein: 6g; Total Carbs: 3g; Fiber: 0g; Net Carbs: 3g; Cholesterol: 111mg

Hardboiled Eggs

Hardboiled eggs are a great source of fat to add to any salad and easy to eat on the go. I make a batch of hardboiled eggs at the start of the week, and my family always goes through them by the weekend.

Prep time | 5 minutes, plus 30 minutes to chill   *Cook time* | 15 minutes

DAIRY-FREE, NUT-FREE, PALEO, VEGETARIAN

Makes 12 eggs

12 large eggs, at room temperature

1. Place the eggs in a single layer in the bottom of a large stockpot. Add cold water to cover the eggs by one inch. Bring to a boil over high heat.

2. Remove the pot from the heat and cover it with the lid. Let sit for 15 minutes.

3. Pour out the hot water, and place the eggs in a large bowl full of ice and water for 30 minutes.

4. Refrigerate.

MAKE AHEAD *Hardboiled eggs can be stored in the refrigerator for up to one week, peeled or unpeeled, in an airtight container.*

MACRONUTRIENTS **62% FAT**, 36% PROTEIN, 2% CARBS

PER SERVING Calories: 144; Total Fat: 10g; Saturated Fat: 3g; Protein: 13g; Total Carbs: 1g; Fiber: 0g; Net Carbs: 1g; Cholesterol: 372mg

Cauliflower Rice

Cauliflower is something I've really grown to love and is my favorite ingredient to experiment with in the kitchen. Cauliflower rice is a perfect replacement any time a dish calls for white rice, brown rice, or couscous. It can also be used as a substitute for mashed potatoes. Serve it raw in salads or, if you prefer it cooked, toss it in a skillet with melted salted butter or olive oil and salt and pepper and cook over medium heat, covered, for 6 to 8 minutes, until tender.

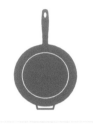

Makes 2 to 3 cups

Prep time | **10 minutes**

DAIRY-FREE, NUT-FREE, EGG-FREE, PALEO, VEGETARIAN, UNDER 30 MINUTES

1 head cauliflower, trimmed

1. Wash and dry the cauliflower, quarter it, and remove any greens. Break the cauliflower apart into large florets.

2. Fill a food processor three-quarters full with florets (you may need to do this step in two or more batches). Pulse until the cauliflower is completely broken down and resembles rice.

3. Serve immediately or cook it if you like.

INGREDIENT TIP *If you don't have a food processor, you can grate the cauliflower on the large holes of a box grater. Many grocery stores also sell fresh or frozen riced cauliflower these days. Look for it in bags in the frozen or refrigerated produce section.*

MACRONUTRIENTS **0% FAT**, 31% PROTEIN, 69% CARBS

PER SERVING (½ cup) Calories: 52; Total Fat: 0g; Saturated Fat: 0g; Protein: 4g; Total Carbs: 10g; Fiber: 5g; Net Carbs: 5g; Cholesterol: 0mg

Zucchini Noodles

When you switch to a low-carb lifestyle, a vegetable spiralizer is well worth the small investment. There are many keto-friendly options for rich, savory, and cheesy dressings and sauces, but without noodles, what are you going to put them on? Low-carb veggies cut into long, spiralized strips make a great noodle replacement and are perfect for soaking up delicious high-fat, low-carb sauces.

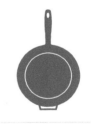

Serves 4

Prep time | 20 minutes   *Cook time* | 10 minutes

DAIRY-FREE, NUT-FREE, EGG-FREE, PALEO, VEGETARIAN, UNDER 30 MINUTES

1 medium zucchini
2 tablespoons salted butter or olive oil
2 garlic cloves, minced
Salt
Freshly ground black pepper

1. Cut the zucchini into strands using a spiralizer, julienne peeler, or knife.

2. In a large skillet over medium-high heat, melt the butter. Add the garlic and cook for 1 to 2 minutes, until the garlic becomes translucent.

3. Add the zucchini strands, and toss to coat them in butter. Cook for 2 to 5 minutes, until crisp-tender.

4. Season with salt and pepper and serve with the sauce and toppings of your choice.

MAKE AHEAD *Store uncooked, spiralized vegetable noodles in a resealable plastic bag or airtight container in the refrigerator for up to 5 days.*

MACRONUTRIENTS **94% FAT**, 1% PROTEIN, 4% CARBS

PER SERVING Calories: 53; Total Fat: 6g; Saturated Fat: 4g; Protein: 0g; Total Carbs: 1g; Fiber: 0g; Net Carbs: 0g; Cholesterol: 15mg

Perfectly Cooked Bacon

Who would have thought you could diet and live a healthy lifestyle with bacon involved? I used to keep bacon out of my diet because of the fat content and all the sodium. Remember uncured, sugar-free bacon is best!

Prep time | 5 minutes   *Cook time* | 20 minutes

DAIRY-FREE, NUT-FREE, EGG-FREE, PALEO, UNDER 30 MINUTES

Serves 8

1 pound uncured bacon slices

1. Preheat the oven to 400°F. Line a sheet pan with aluminum foil for easy cleanup.

2. Arrange the bacon slices in a single layer on the prepared sheet pan.

3. Bake for 12 to 20 minutes, depending on the thickness of the bacon and how crispy you like it.

4. Transfer the cooked bacon to a paper towel–lined plate to drain.

5. Serve hot with your favorite meal or store in an airtight container in the refrigerator for up to 5 days.

VARIATION TIP *You can also cook bacon on the stovetop. Start with a cold skillet (cast iron preferred) and arrange the bacon slices in a single layer in the bottom. Cook on low for 8 to 12 minutes, or to your desired crispiness.*

MACRONUTRIENTS **74% FAT**, 26% PROTEIN, 0% CARBS

PER SERVING (2 slices) Calories: 110; Total Fat: 9g; Saturated Fat: 4g; Protein: 7g; Total Carbs: 0g; Fiber: 0g; Net Carbs: 0g; Cholesterol: 20mg

Salsa Shredded Chicken

This recipe, eaten on its own as a meal, is not keto, but it is a great basic recipe that can be used as a starting point for many meals that are. It's an easy way to prepare chicken so you'll have it on hand when you need a quick dinner. This will undoubtedly help you stay on track with your keto goals.

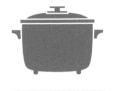

Serves 8

Prep time | 5 minutes   *Cook time* | 6 to 8 hours

DAIRY-FREE, NUT-FREE, EGG-FREE, PALEO

Olive oil cooking spray (optional)

8 boneless, skinless chicken breasts

2 cups salsa

2 teaspoons ground cumin

2 tablespoons garlic powder

Juice of 2 limes

Salt

Freshly ground black pepper

1. Spray a slow cooker with the cooking spray or line it with a slow-cooker liner.

2. Place the chicken breasts in the prepared slow cooker. Add the salsa, cumin, garlic powder, and lime juice, and season with salt and pepper. Cover and cook on low for 6 to 8 hours.

3. Remove the chicken breasts from the slow cooker and shred using two forks. Return the shredded chicken to the slow cooker with the leftover juices, and stir until combined.

4. Serve immediately or store for up to 5 days refrigerated in an airtight container.

MACRONUTRIENTS **23% FAT,** 63% PROTEIN, 14% CARBS

PER SERVING Calories: 168; Total Fat: 4g; Saturated Fat: 2g; Protein: 26g; Total Carbs: 6g; Fiber: 1g; Net Carbs: 5g; Cholesterol: 65mg

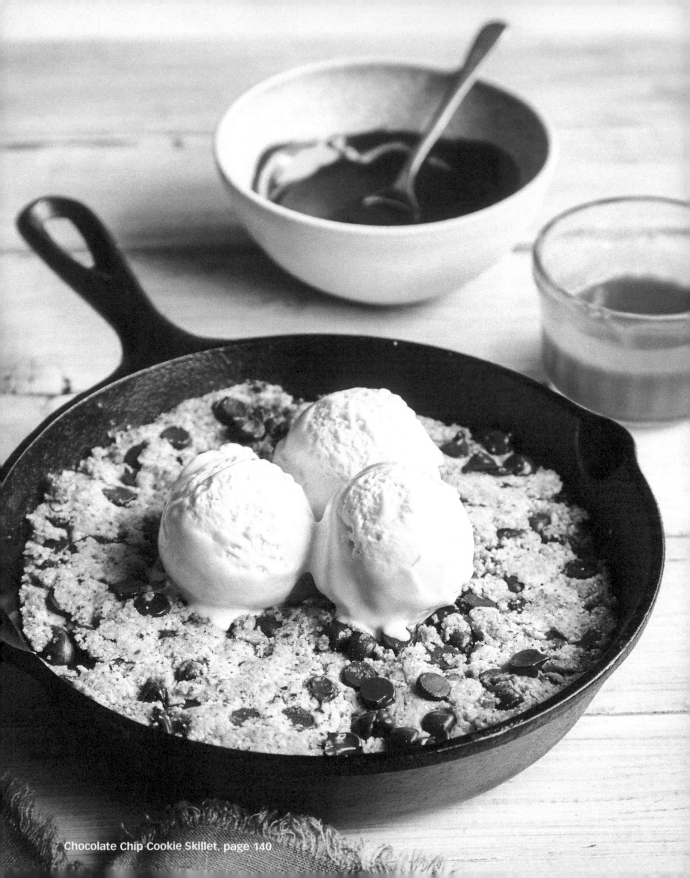

Chocolate Chip Cookie Skillet, page 140

CHAPTER 10 | SWEETS

Raspberry Cheesecake Fluff

Craving something sweet? This decadent Raspberry Cheesecake Fluff will do the trick and leave you guilt-free! You can also use this fluff to top any warm mug cake, keto-approved cheesecake, or a fresh bowl of berries.

Prep time | 5 minutes

NUT-FREE, EGG-FREE, UNDER 30 MINUTES

Serves 4

1 cup heavy (whipping) cream

8 ounces cream cheese, at room temperature

4 ounces raspberries

½ cup sugar substitute (such as Swerve)

1 teaspoon vanilla extract

Pinch salt

1. In blender or in a bowl using a hand mixer, whip the cream to stiff peaks, 2 to 4 minutes.

2. Add the cream cheese, raspberries, sugar substitute, vanilla, and salt, and blend until smooth and well combined.

MACRONUTRIENTS **88% FAT,** 5% PROTEIN, 7% CARBS

PER SERVING Calories: 417; Total Fat: 41g; Saturated Fat: 25g; Protein: 5g; Total Carbs: 7g; Fiber: 2g; Net Carbs: 5g; Cholesterol: 143mg

Keto Hot Fudge

When you're not pairing this hot fudge up with sugar-free whipped cream and adding it to your favorite low-carb ice cream or the Chocolate Chip Cookie Skillet (page 140), you will probably find yourself eating it right from the jar, and that's okay! You can store it refrigerated in a mason jar for up to a week—if it lasts that long.

Serves 10

Prep time | 5 minutes   *Cook time* | 10 minutes

NUT-FREE, EGG-FREE, VEGETARIAN, UNDER 30 MINUTES

½ cup (1 stick) salted butter

4 ounces dark chocolate
   (85% or higher)

2 tablespoons unsweetened
   cocoa powder

1 cup sugar substitute (such as Swerve)

1 cup heavy (whipping) cream

2 teaspoons vanilla extract

Pinch salt

1. In a medium saucepan over medium heat, melt the butter and chocolate. Add the cocoa powder and sweetener, and whisk until the powder and sweetener dissolve, 3 to 5 minutes.

2. Add the cream and bring to a boil, stirring constantly. Reduce the heat to low, and add the vanilla and salt.

3. Remove from the heat, let rest for 5 minutes, and serve hot over your favorite dessert.

MACRONUTRIENTS **91% FAT**, 3% PROTEIN, 6% CARBS

PER SERVING Calories: 237; Total Fat: 24g; Saturated Fat: 14g; Protein: 2g; Total Carbs: 5g; Fiber: 2g; Net Carbs: 3g; Cholesterol: 57mg

Hot Caramel Sauce

It's always nice to have dessert sauces like this on hand. A spoon and a quick trip to the fridge will curb any sweet cravings. It also cuts down on time when prepping recipes like the Caramel Almond Bars (page 143).

Prep time | 5 minutes   *Cook time* | 10 minutes

Serves 8

NUT-FREE, VEGETARIAN, UNDER 30 MINUTES

½ cup (1 stick) salted butter

¼ cup sugar substitute (such as Swerve)

1 cup heavy (whipping) cream

¼ to ½ teaspoon xanthan gum

½ teaspoon salt

1. In a large saucepan over medium-low heat, melt the butter. Whisk in the sugar substitute until it is dissolved and incorporated, 3 to 5 minutes.

2. Add the cream, xanthan gum, and salt to the mixture, whisking continuously. Bring to a boil and let boil for 1 minute, then remove from the heat.

3. Serve hot.

MAKE AHEAD *Make this sauce up to 5 days in advance. Let it cool to room temperature before putting in a covered storage container and storing in the refrigerator.*

MACRONUTRIENTS **98% FAT**, 1% PROTEIN, 1% CARBS

PER SERVING Calories: 202; Total Fat: 22g; Saturated Fat: 14g; Protein: 1g; Total Carbs: 1g; Fiber: 0g; Net Carbs: 1g; Cholesterol: 71mg

5-Minute Chocolate Mousse

You'd never guess this fluffy, whipped dessert was sugar-free or dairy-free! Full-fat coconut cream is a healthy, dairy-free alternative to heavy whipping cream. I love the flavor it adds to shakes, curries, soups, and ice cream. Here it makes for a rich and chocolatey mousse.

Prep time | **5 minutes**

Serves 4

DAIRY-FREE, NUT-FREE, EGG-FREE, PALEO, VEGETARIAN, UNDER 30 MINUTES

1 (14-ounce) can coconut cream, chilled

3 tablespoons unsweetened cocoa powder

¼ cup sugar substitute (such as Swerve)

1 teaspoon vanilla extract

1. In a large mixing bowl, whip the coconut cream with a hand mixer until fluffy, about 3 minutes. If you don't have a hand mixer, you can whip it in the blender.

2. Fold in the cocoa powder, sugar substitute, and vanilla and serve immediately.

VARIATION TIP *Add half a ripe avocado to make the mousse even creamier!*

MACRONUTRIENTS **89% FAT**, 2% PROTEIN, 9% CARBS

PER SERVING Calories: 222; Total Fat: 22g; Saturated Fat: 21g; Protein: 1g; Total Carbs: 5g; Fiber: 1g; Net Carbs: 4g; Cholesterol: 0mg

Pumpkin Mousse

We don't wait for autumn to break out the pumpkin pie spice. We enjoy it all year long at our house. We love it in this satisfying, creamy pumpkin mousse. Pumpkin pie spice is a great thing to keep in your spice cabinet. You can add it to your favorite keto latte, roasted vegetables, and pancake recipe. If you don't have pumpkin pie spice on hand, try substituting with ground nutmeg, cloves, or cinnamon.

Serves 4

Prep time | **10 minutes, plus 30 minutes to chill**

NUT-FREE, EGG-FREE, VEGETARIAN

8 ounces cream cheese, at
    room temperature
1 cup canned pumpkin purée
1 cup heavy (whipping) cream
2 tablespoons sugar substitute
    (such as Swerve)
1 teaspoon vanilla extract
1 teaspoon pumpkin pie spice
½ teaspoon ground cinnamon

1. In a large mixer or in a large bowl with a hand mixer, cream together the cream cheese and pumpkin until smooth, 1 to 2 minutes. If you don't have either type of mixer, you can use a blender.

2. Add the cream, sweetener, vanilla, pumpkin pie spice, and cinnamon. Mix on high for 3 to 5 minutes, or until fluffy.

3. Chill for 30 minutes before serving.

INGREDIENT TIP *Make sure not to purchase pumpkin pie filling, and watch for added sugar in the pumpkin purée.*

MACRONUTRIENTS **88% FAT,** 5% PROTEIN, 7% CARBS

PER SERVING Calories: 419; Total Fat: 41g; Saturated Fat: 25g; Protein: 6g; Total Carbs: 9g; Fiber: 3g; Net Carbs: 6g; Cholesterol: 144mg

Snickerdoodle Mug Cake

Think of those fresh-out-of-the-oven, gooey cinnamon snickerdoodle cookies in mug cake form. This is dangerously quick to make and will fill your house with the smell of freshly baked cinnamon cookies. This is a calorically dense cake, so although it is made in one mug, note that the recipe serves 2, so you'll have to share!

Serves 2

Prep time | 5 minutes   *Cook time* | 2 minutes

VEGETARIAN, UNDER 30 MINUTES

2 tablespoons salted butter

2 tablespoons sugar substitute
   (such as Swerve)

2 tablespoons almond flour

2 tablespoons heavy (whipping) cream
   or coconut cream

1 large egg

1 teaspoon ground cinnamon,
   plus more for serving

½ teaspoon vanilla extract

½ teaspoon baking powder

¼ teaspoon cream of tartar

¼ teaspoon salt (optional)

Cinnamon, for sprinkling

1. In a coffee mug or glass measuring cup, microwave the butter until melted, about 30 seconds. Add the sugar substitute and stir vigorously with a fork. Add the almond flour, cream, egg, cinnamon, vanilla, baking powder, cream of tartar, and salt (if using), and mix until everything is combined.

2. Microwave for 50 to 70 seconds, or until the middle of the cake is moist, being careful to not overcook.

3. Sprinkle with cinnamon and serve.

VARIATION TIP *Instead of including the cream in the batter before microwaving, add it over the top when you're ready to eat it.*

MACRONUTRIENTS **90% FAT,** 8% PROTEIN, 2% CARBS

PER SERVING Calories: 229; Total Fat: 23g; Saturated Fat: 12g; Protein: 5g; Total Carbs: 2g; Fiber: 1g; Net Carbs: 1g; Cholesterol: 145mg

Chocolate Chip Cookie Skillet

On special occasions, it's fun to serve dessert right from the skillet. Just top with your favorite low-carb ice cream, Hot Caramel Sauce (page 136), and Keto Hot Fudge (page 135).

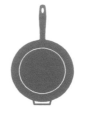

Prep time | 10 minutes, plus 10 minutes to rest   *Cook time* | 25 minutes

DAIRY-FREE, VEGETARIAN

Serves 8

Olive oil cooking spray or coconut oil,
  for preparing the skillet
1 cup almond flour
½ cup coconut flour
½ teaspoon baking soda
1 teaspoon salt
½ cup coconut oil, at room temperature
¼ cup sugar substitute
  (such as Swerve)
1 large egg
1 teaspoon vanilla extract
1 cup sugar-free chocolate chips

1. Preheat the oven to 350°F. Spray a 9-inch cast iron skillet, pie dish, or cake pan with cooking spray or grease it with coconut oil.

2. In a large bowl, whisk together the almond flour, coconut flour, baking soda, and salt. Add the coconut oil, sugar substitute, egg, and vanilla, and whisk until combined. Fold in the chocolate chips.

3. Pour the batter into the prepared skillet and bake for 20 to 25 minutes, or until brown on the edges and gooey in the center.

4. Let rest for 5 to 10 minutes and serve warm.

VARIATION TIP *Add your favorite nuts to the batter before baking. Chopped macadamia nuts, cashews, and pecans work best.*

MACRONUTRIENTS **69% FAT**, 7% PROTEIN, 24% CARBS

PER SERVING Calories: 390; Total Fat: 30g; Saturated Fat: 19g; Protein: 7g; Total Carbs: 25g; Fiber: 5g; Net Carbs: 20g; Cholesterol: 33mg

Peanut Butter Fat Bombs

We're used to worrying about too much fat in our diets, and now that you are low-carb we want to make sure you are getting enough! As you transition into your low-carb lifestyle, fat bombs are a great way to increase healthy fats and keep you satisfied.

Prep time | 15 minutes, plus at least 4 hours to freeze
Cook time | 1 minute

EGG-FREE, VEGETARIAN

Serves 10

2 tablespoons coconut oil

2 tablespoons salted butter

¼ cup peanut butter

¼ cup sugar substitute (such as Swerve)

2 teaspoons vanilla extract

2 tablespoons cream cheese

1. In a medium microwave-safe bowl, combine the coconut oil, butter, peanut butter, sugar substitute, vanilla, and cream cheese. Microwave in 15-second increments, stirring in between, until everything is melted and combined.

2. Pour the mixture into an ice cube tray or mini cupcake pan, and freeze for at least 4 hours.

3. Remove from the molds and store in an airtight container or a resealable plastic bag in the freezer for up to 3 months.

VARIATION TIP *If you have leftover chocolate chips from making the Chocolate Chip Cookie Skillet (page 140), this is a great recipe to add them to.*

MACRONUTRIENTS 86% FAT, 8% PROTEIN, 6% CARBS

PER SERVING Calories: 94; Total Fat: 9g; Saturated Fat: 5g; Protein: 2g; Total Carbs: 1g; Fiber: 0g; Net Carbs: 0g; Cholesterol: 9mg

Key-Lime Cheesecake Cups

These tart cheesecake cups are a perfect addition to any get-together or gathering. They will keep the non-low-carb guests asking for seconds and questioning whether the ketogenic lifestyle might just be for them after all.

Prep time | 10 minutes   *Cook time* | 30 minutes

VEGETARIAN

Serves 12

FOR THE CRUST

1 cup raw almonds

½ cup (1 stick) salted butter, melted

2 tablespoons sugar substitute
(such as Swerve)

FOR THE FILLING

2 (8-ounce) packages cream cheese,
at room temperature

2 large eggs

½ cup sugar substitute
(such as Swerve)

2 limes, juiced and zested

2 teaspoons vanilla extract

Preheat the oven to 375°F. Line a muffin tin with paper liners.

TO MAKE THE CRUST

1. In a blender, pulse the almonds until finely ground. Add the butter and sweetener, and mix until combined.

2. Press the crust mixture into the bottom of the cups, dividing it equally.

3. Bake for 5 minutes.

TO MAKE THE FILLING AND BAKE

4. In a blender, blend to combine the cream cheese, eggs, sweetener, lime juice, lime zest, and vanilla.

5. Evenly divide the filling, spooning it over the parbaked crusts. Bake for 15 to 20 minutes, or until the cheesecake is cooked through.

6. Let rest and refrigerate for at least an hour, or until firm. Serve cold.

VARIATION TIP *If key lime isn't your flavor of choice, leave out the lime and replace with berries or enjoy classic cheesecake.*

MACRONUTRIENTS **87% FAT,** 7% PROTEIN, 6% CARBS

PER SERVING Calories: 279; Total Fat: 27g; Saturated Fat: 13g; Protein: 6g; Total Carbs: 4g; Fiber: 2g; Net Carbs: 2g; Cholesterol: 93mg

Caramel Almond Bars

These grain-free, gooey bars will leave you feeling like you aren't on a diet at all. The crumbly, flaky texture will have you licking your fingers and rescuing every dropped crumb.

Prep time | 10 minutes, plus 10 minutes to rest   *Cook time* | 20 minutes

EGG-FREE, VEGETARIAN

Serves 12

6 tablespoons salted butter, melted, plus more for preparing the dish

1 cup unsweetened flaked coconut

1 cup sliced almonds

¾ cup almond flour

½ cup sugar substitute (such as Swerve)

1 teaspoon salt

½ teaspoon baking soda

1 cup sugar-free chocolate chips

1 cup Hot Caramel Sauce (page 136) (optional)

1. Preheat the oven to 350°F. Grease a square baking dish with butter.

2. In a food processor, combine the coconut, almonds, almond flour, sugar substitute, salt, baking soda, and 6 tablespoons melted butter, and pulse until crumbly. Fold in the chocolate chips, and press the batter into the prepared baking dish.

3. Bake for 15 to 20 minutes, or until golden brown.

4. Pour the caramel sauce (if using) over the bars and let rest for 10 minutes.

5. Serve warm.

MAKE IT PALEO *Substitute coconut oil for the butter and skip the caramel sauce.*

MACRONUTRIENTS 83% FAT, 7% PROTEIN, 10% CARBS

PER SERVING Calories: 229; Total Fat: 21g; Saturated Fat: 10g; Protein: 4g; Total Carbs: 6g; Fiber: 3g; Net Carbs: 3g; Cholesterol: 15mg

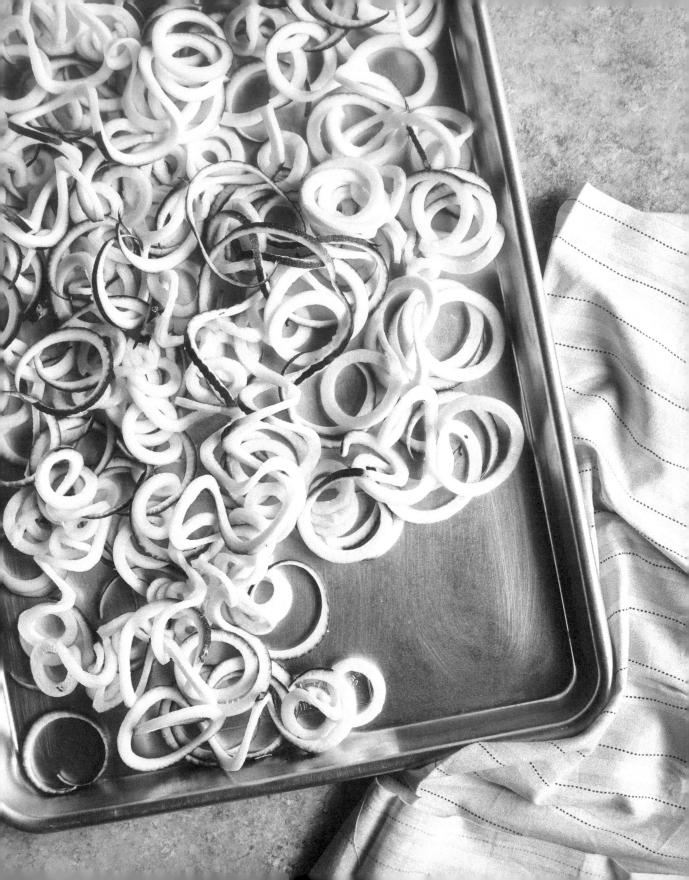

MEASUREMENTS

VOLUME EQUIVALENTS (Liquid)

US Standard (ounces)	US Standard (approximate)	Metric
2 tablespoons	1 fl. oz.	30 mL
¼ cup	2 fl. oz.	60 mL
½ cup	4 fl. oz.	120 mL
1 cup	8 fl. oz.	240 mL
1½ cups	12 fl. oz	355 mL
2 cups or 1 pint	16 fl. oz.	475 mL
4 cups or 1 quart	32 fl. oz.	1 L
1 gallon	128 fl. oz.	4 L

OVEN TEMPERATURES

Fahrenheit (F)	Celsius (C) (approximate)
250°F	120°C
300°F	150°C
325°F	165°C
350°F	180°C
375°F	190°C
400°F	200°C
425°F	220°C
450°F	230°C

VOLUME EQUIVALENTS (Dry)

US Standard	Metric (approximate)
⅛ teaspoon	0.5 mL
¼ teaspoon	1 mL
½ teaspoon	2 mL
¾ teaspoon	4 mL
1 teaspoon	5 mL
1 tablespoon	15 mL
¼ cup	59 mL
⅓ cup	79 mL
½ cup	118 mL
⅔ cup	156 mL
¾ cup	177 mL
1 cup	235 mL
2 cups or 1 pint	475 mL
3 cups	700 mL
4 cups or 1 quart	1 L

WEIGHT EQUIVALENTS

US Standard	Metric (approximate)
½ ounce	15 g
1 ounce	30 g
2 ounces	60 g
4 ounces	115 g
8 ounces	225 g
12 ounces	340 g
16 ounces or 1 pound	455 g

RESOURCES

Below are a few resources that have played a huge role in my own ketogenic journey.

Websites and Blogs

ruledme.com

dietdoctor.com

pinterest.com

mariamindbodyhealth.com

ketodietapp.com

healthfulpursuit.com

fitketogirls.com

Keto Macro Calculators

ruled.me/keto-calculator

ketoconnect.net/calculator

Apps

My Fitness Pal (for macro tracking)

Podcasts

The Keto Diet Podcast

Livin' La Vida Low Carb

The Ketogenic Athlete

Fat-Burning Man

2 Keto Dudes

The Tim Ferriss Show

Books

The Keto Diet by Leanne Vogel

Keto Clarity by Jimmy Moore & Eric Westman

The Ketogenic Bible by Dr. Jacob Wilson & Ryan Lowery

RECIPE INDEX

INDEX

ACKNOWLEDGMENTS

I'm genuinely grateful for the amount of support I received in creating and writing this cookbook. Without the love from my family and friends, it wouldn't have come together like it did.

Thank you to my husband, for his encouragement to stay true to myself, his endless support, and his desire for me to find what makes me happy. He experienced what single fatherhood would look like while I wrote this book, and also washed countless dishes after I worked—or played—in the kitchen.

And to my beautiful Gracie Rose. I did this for you, baby girl. You inspire me and I want to be all I can for you.

I want to thank my dad for his eclectic taste and passion for cooking. Watching his love in the kitchen is what led me to find my own passion for creating in the kitchen.

Thank you to my sweet mother for her creative gene and her ability to create magical memories around the dinner table.

Thank you to my editor Talia Platz and the team at Callisto Media. So much went on behind the scenes, and they were so great to work with, guiding this first-time author through the publishing process. Thanks to Brandy and Toni for believing in me and pushing me to new limits.

Thanks to my family at 7K Fit, you have been so welcoming and supportive of my little family and our move to Evanston. Each of you inspire us on the daily and have made our dreams come true.

To Jane, who lit my fire for keto, and was the other half of Fit Keto Girls. And to Liz, whose genius guided me to find the power of one through social media.

That connection brought me the online ketogenic community, to whom I offer my greatest thanks. Without the support from my Instagram followers, Facebook group members, and the wonderful friends I have met, this opportunity simply would not have happened. Your stories, examples, and ketogenic transformations inspire me. Because of you I am passionate about sharing the tools, recipes, and inspiration that all of us can gain through living a ketogenic lifestyle.

Thank you to every one of you who provided encouragement, offered input, inspired the recipes, and brought this book to life.

To you the reader, I hope you discover the positive difference this can make in your life, and in the lives of those you love.

ABOUT THE AUTHOR

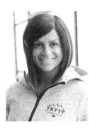 **Liz Williams** has devoted her career to helping others stay fit and feel good on the ketogenic diet. As a cofounder of the ketogenic lifestyle blog *Fit Keto Girls*, Liz is strongly committed to promoting health and wellness. She also shares her experiences with the ketogenic diet on her popular Instagram handle @ thefittrainerswife. She lives in Evanston, Wyoming, with her daughter and husband. Learn more at FitKetoGirls.com.